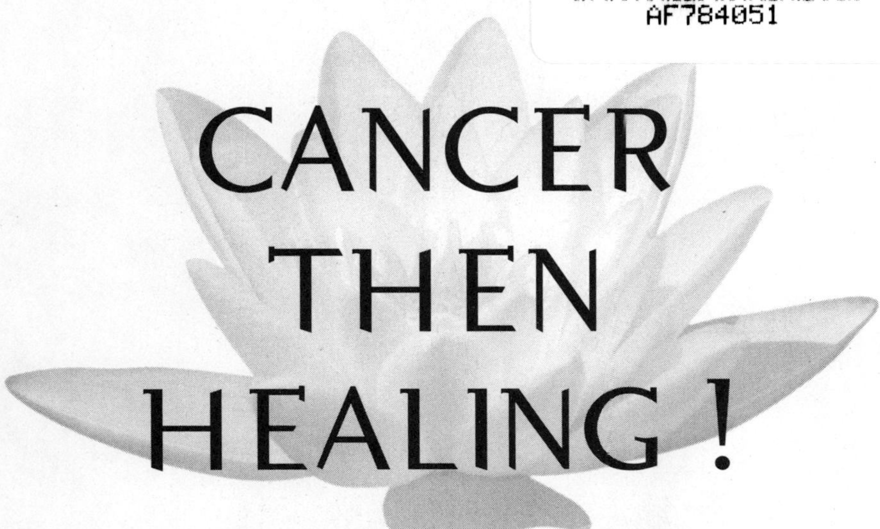

CANCER THEN HEALING!

15 DECISIONS TO MAKE WHEN YOU OR A LOVED ONE ARE TOLD "YOU HAVE CANCER" OR ANY LIFE-THREATENING DISEASE

STRAY DOG PRESS

CANCER THEN HEALING

15 DECISIONS TO MAKE

WHEN YOU OR A LOVED ONE ARE TOLD

"YOU HAVE CANCER" OR ANY LIFE THREATENING DISEASE.

BY MICKI VOISARD

Published by:

STRAY DOG PRESS

P.O. Box 1099

Calistoga, CA. 94515 USA

First Printing 1998

Printed in the United States of America

DEDICATION

TO ALL WOMEN AND MEN AND THEIR FAMILIES WHO HAVE SHARED THEIR WORST "WINTERS" WITH ME.

TO MY HUSBAND DAVID, WHO HELPED ME FIND MY WAY IN A "BLINDING SNOW STORM".

ACKNOWLEDGEMENT

I would like to thank my husband David, for his undying support. My three dogs - Otis, Dandy and Hannah for reminding me when it was time to take a walk. My six cats for not jumping on my keyboard too much. The other fine people who need to be recognized are Walter and Lorraine Arnold, Sandra and Jackson Carr, Lelain Crist, Nancy Eckberg, Phil and Michael Franklin, Ann Hill, Dorothy Kingren, Sparky Kramer, Paul Meland, Jim Miller, Rosemary Montilla, Ann Procter, Maureen Redl, Joan Reed, China Roberson, Liza Russ, Jeanne Sayner, Jean and Bernie Slingerland, Thomas Smith, Charlie Spillar, Fran Spratt, Jeanette Stedifor, Jane and Paul Voisard, Jody and Jeff Wheaton, and Don Yates.

Also for: Copyediting by Carolynne Gamble
Layout by Dan Yazvac, D.A.Y.Graphics
Cover Design by Kathi Dunn, Dunn and Associates
Back Cover Copy by Susan Kendrick

INTRODUCTION

IN THE MIDST OF WINTER I FINALLY LEARNED THAT THERE WAS WITHIN ME AN INVINCIBLE SUMMER.

- ALBERT CAMUS

Rattlesnakes know when to strike. I know, I have lived among them for over fifteen years. I have been bitten by them, had them in my house, in my car and watched their secret "combat dance". When rattlesnakes strike, they usually give you only one fang full of venom. They just want you out of their way and are smart not to waste the other fang of venom. That is saved for another attack.

This is not a book on rattlesnakes. This is a book on **healing from cancer.** Some people might think I am making a comparison between rattlesnakes and cancer. No way. I have far too much respect for these reptiles. Such patient, cunning, tenacious creatures have taught me a lot about transmutation and hunting prey. I have been told by Native Americans that since I have been bitten by a rattlesnake, I have "snake medicine". With snake medicine comes the ability to transmute, to change forms.

Cancer is one form I have transmuted. I am not alone in my ability to change. You will read about many other people who did the same, and they have not been bitten by a rattlesnake. Each one found personal tenacity, practiced patience and became cunning. In the four years since I was "transmuted", I have interviewed over 500 people who have called me for suggestions for alternative treatments of cancer.

Some people had already used conventional medicine, others had just been diagnosed, and the rest were determined to find some alternative way they could heal themselves.

Each one told me a different story with a similar theme. They were not going to listen to one opinion and they knew they had options. They may not have known about their options right away, but once they hunted them down, they became tenacious.

Changing from one form to another takes time. It also requires help from your environment and tremendous focus. When a rattlesnake goes through transmutation, or shedding its skin, it is very weak. His eyes cover with a thin layer of skin and his eyesight is diminished. He strikes at anything since he knows he can not totally depend on other senses. He needs the help of rocks to break off the old layers of skin. If the snake is not healthy, he will not survive this long ordeal. This is a perfect time for predators to catch him at his most vulnerable time. When he strikes, he will not clearly see what it is he has struck at, until it is too late.

Maybe you do not appreciate rattlesnakes at all, or they scare you more than any wild creature. My heart has skipped many beats when I have heard their frightful rattle. Still, I hope you will take on the qualities of "snake medicine" and learn what you are capable of changing in your life, when you are faced with a life- threatening disease.

Like the rattlesnake going through transmutation, you are at your most vulnerable point in life. Learning you have cancer, dulls your senses and makes most of us retreat in fear.

Chapter One outlines the 15 Decisions that were compiled from conversations with 500 people who shared their stories with me. These 15 Decisions helped people move from fear to healing.

Chapter Two tells my tale, my personal experience with cancer. **When** I found my "snake medicine" and **How** I used it.

Chapter Three starts a more detailed explanation of the 15 Decisions, with each Decision being allotted its own chapter.

Even if you are reading this book three, six, or twelve months after your diagnosis, it is never too late to focus on your healing!

I firmly believe that you will feel more hopeful after reading these 15 Decisions. There are no guarantees, but the encouraging news is that the "winters" are getting shorter and, for some, easier. After talking personally and publicly with hundreds of women and men, I am excited to tell you that more people are experiencing the "spring" after the "winter" of cancer.

You do not have to be bitten by a rattlesnake to learn to shed your skin. There are many books offering the hope and courage you need to endure. This is where courage is born - accepting responsibility when you answer two crucial questions: "Whose life is this anyway?" and "Who is in charge here?" It is your life - LEARN TO HEAL WITH IT !

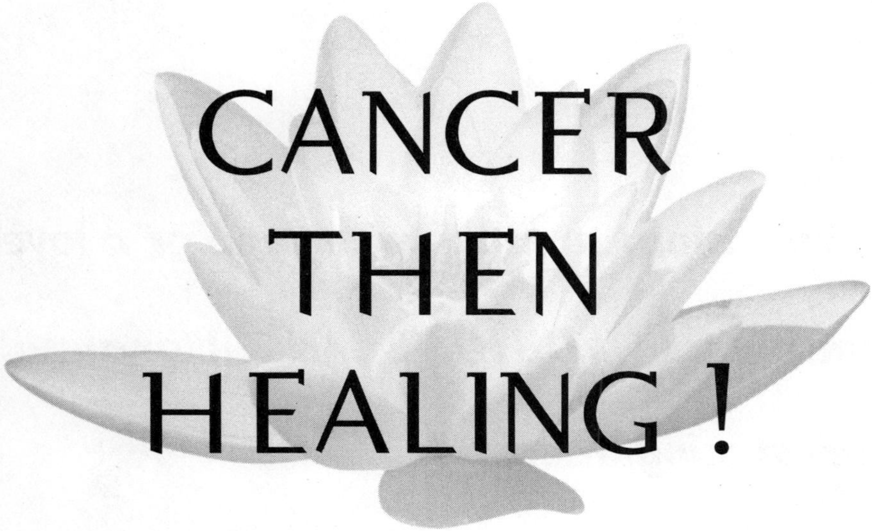

CANCER THEN HEALING!

15 DECISIONS TO MAKE WHEN YOU OR A LOVED ONE ARE TOLD "YOU HAVE CANCER" OR ANY LIFE-THREATENING DISEASE

15 Decisions to make when you or a loved one are told "YOU HAVE CANCER" or any life threatening disease.

CHAPTER ONE

1. **DECIDE** within the first fifteen minutes if you want to overcome this disease or not. This seems obvious, but it is rarely considered until the shock wears off. Make this your priority. **FOCUS IMMEDIATELY ON HEALING.**
2. Pay attention to your breathing. Take long, slow, deep breaths. Calm yourself as much as possible - **DO NOT ALLOW THIS NEWS TO OVERWHELM YOU!**
3. The words **"CANCER"** and **"AIDS"** have a profound and powerful effect on our society. Turn it around. Replace your thinking with words that propel you to action. Call on your **PERSONAL POWER** often. Learn to use it.
4. Do not ask, "How long do I have?". Your doctor can only give you a scientific generalization. **YOU ARE A UNIQUE INDIVIDUAL**; your immune system is unique.
5. Do not commit to any procedure or treatment for at least 24 hours, preferably longer. Give yourself time alone to think or meditate. Go away somewhere for a day or overnight. **THERE ARE MANY ALTERNATIVES,** even if one alternative is to do nothing for the time being.
6. **CONSIDER ALL OPTIONS.** You are like a hub in a wheel. The spokes are the people and treatments that will be helping you. Your doctor is only one of those spokes.

7. When you are alone, **REFOCUS YOUR THOUGHTS.** Align with great ideas to use when fear returns. Stop analyzing. Give yourself some downtime. This is where courage is born!
8. Cancer promotes change. **START YOUR TRANSFORM-ATION** now.
9. Make yourself **LAUGH** before you cry.
10. Fill your hospital room or home with **FUN**, whimsical **ART**, or pictures from a magazine of places where your mind can go when you need strength.
11. Do not allow anyone to tell you that you are in denial. **YOU ARE IN REALITY!**
12. Using war terminology to describe a disease or how you are dealing with it, is not healing. Diseases take time to heal and one cannot sustain a "battle" for very long. Say **"I AM HEALING!"**
13. Attitude is very important. Back up your **ATTITUDE WITH ACTION!**
14. Believe in yourself and your decisions. **YOU ARE RIGHT!**
15. Treating Cancer is your business. **HEAL WITH IT!**

NO WIMPY WOMEN HERE

CHAPTER TWO

"I don't want to be a wimpy woman!" Lisa told me emphatically. Her voice had a touch of pleading, but I believed her from my heart. Never having seen or met her, I knew only what she talked about and how she sounded over the telephone.

I have talked with over five hundred women and men about ovarian cancer or other cancers. Lisa is the one who keeps me answering my phone. Her strength and innocence made her very appealing. She was 22 years old, in her last semester of graduate school, and taking her finals when her life was to change forever and soon come to an end.

Recently separated from her husband of two years, the last thing Lisa needed in her life was persistent and agonizing back pain. She had a very difficult time sitting in class, and walking around campus was pure torture. Strange, she thought, because she was the most athletic girl in her family of five girls and two boys. She attributed her pain to the constant stress in her life. Now, for the first time, she had felt a cyst near her left ovary, obvious by just feeling her stomach.

With access to the Internet, she spent hours researching her pain. What she found alarmed her, and she decided to return to her gynecologist for the fourth time in one year.

At her gynecologist's office, Lisa felt the same frustration she had encountered on the previous three visits. He rebuked and ridiculed any information she had researched on the Internet. Lisa did not back off and insisted on another sonogram, her third one in a year. Her doctor did the sonogram reluctantly and found nothing. She brought up her research once again explaining to him that she thought her symptoms resembled those of ovarian cancer. "Only women over sixty get ovarian cancer," he replied.

The doctor suggested she finish her finals and take a few weeks off to recuperate. Defeated, Lisa went home to prepare for her finals.

Still dealing with pain and feeling very uncomfortable eating or going to the bathroom, Lisa barely made it to her first final. Feeling nauseous, flushed and tired by the second hour of her testing, she felt a severe cramping sensation in her abdomen. Within minutes she passed out in class and awoke in the hospital with her husband and parents surrounding her bed.

She found she was hooked up to an IV and was told she had undergone emergency surgery. She was frightened and confused and her husband went on to tell her the worst of the news.

The cyst she had been so concerned about was an ovarian tumor. It had burst during her final exam, filling her body with cancer cells. Her future was bleak and not even chemotherapy was recommended.

In April, Lisa moved back in with her husband because she needed his insurance, and he offered his support. Lisa called me in October. Within seven months she now had a brain and lung tumor which caused labored breathing and memory lapses.

In our first conversation, Lisa was angry, but her sense of humor was ever present. She felt grateful that for at least five months she felt well enough to do things she always wanted to do. Still living with her husband, but more as a friend, she saw no reason to reconcile their marriage. She thought it would be easier for him after she was gone.

We talked four more times until just after Christmas. I thought of her and gave her a call. Several times I got their answering machine before I finally connected with her husband. Lisa died three days after Christmas. Not wanting to return to the hospital she stayed at home. The last few days were agonizing, but in a whispered voice she would continually say, "I don't want to be a wimpy woman."

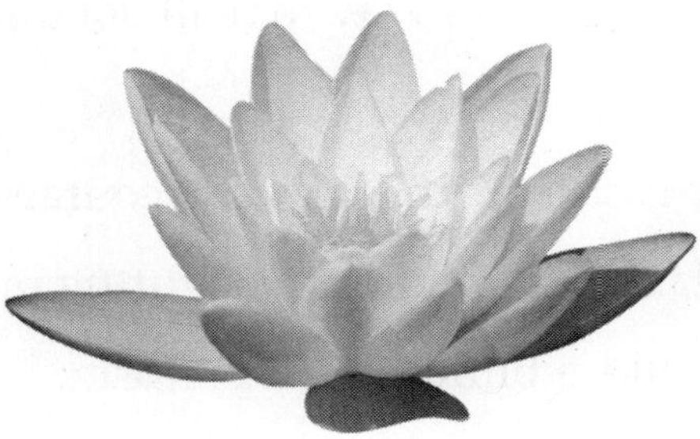

I have seldom talked with anyone whose cancer was as advanced as Lisa's. Most women I talk with are between Stages 2 to 3c, with an occasional Stage 4, like Lisa's. The incredible thing is that a misdiagnosis like Lisa's is repeated in case after case. The symptoms are identical and, in my mind, dangerously obvious.

Are doctors just not hearing? Do all women who come into a gynecologist's office complain of the same symptoms? Does it matter if the doctor is a man or would a woman doctor be more responsive?

Less than half the women I interviewed had women doctors, including myself. The decisions rest in our lap. Our health is our business, but we have been raised to believe doctors give us health. We give them money, they give us a cure.

Lisa was a Harvard graduate student with an exceptional IQ. She even possessed the ability to research her own problem. It is easy to understand how Lisa was defeated each time she went back to her gynecologist. One important factor eludes us. Lisa was sick and in terrible pain. She listened to her doctor and went where her insurance would pay for treatment. This led her down the wrong path. This is not to say that all doctors lead you down the wrong path.

My own story is similar to Lisa's but courage hatched in me before it was too late. I spent months fighting my way out of the system and it was like a blinding snow storm.

FOR WHOM THE BELL TOLLS

A return trip home from Atlanta, Georgia was the first time I remember hearing the "bell" toll loudly. It came in the form of pain - persistent, agonizing pain. That pain stayed for two years until it was finally evicted through surgery and the removal of the tumor. This was really the final warning, but at the time I thought it was an early signal. Somehow I never "heard" those other bells. The pain moved in like an unwanted roommate, and had a bad influence on my behavior. It sent me on a wild goose chase that nearly cost me my life.

For two years, I spent a lot of time reading magazines in the waiting rooms of many doctors and practitioners. I thought they might be able to help me. What I really needed to do was stop, collect my thoughts and clear my mind.

This was not Hollywood; this was real life. As anyone who knows agonizing pain, clearing one's mind is the impossible dream. So the two stroll together - the pain and the unclear mind - the odd couple rooming in one's body.

In those two agonizing years when I thought I was receiving an "early warning" signal, I saw four gynecologists, two for several visits. Each one gave me a physical exam and a pap smear. I also had three sonograms. The doctors agreed on the same diagnosis - an extremely large fibroid tumor located either on my uterus or on my left ovary. Each one gave me their vote of confidence. There was nothing to be concerned about. Each believed that as soon as I started menopause, the fibroid would shrink. I was 43 years old at the time. According to each gynecologist, I was a prime suspect for early menopause. Case dismissed.

The "final warning" was constant and agonizing back pain. I had tolerated occasional back pain for years before this. In fact, I had tolerated many problems before the last bell tolled, but I ignored them. I was told by doctors and others that I "looked the picture of health." I believed it myself and could not believe anything else. Meanwhile, inside my body, the symptoms grew.

Symptoms for ovarian cancer vary until the late stages. Many are the same as pre-menopausal symptoms.

In conversations and interviews with hundreds of people who have had cancer, many of us have similar problems. Back problems do occur from many cancers. In my case, the tumor was resting on my pelvic bone and pinching the 5th vertebra. This caused the sciatic nerve in my right side to be constantly inflamed from the weight of the tumor. My spinal cord was totally out of whack, pulling on my neck, and causing constant headaches and sinus problems. My shoulders were always sore and my arms and hands were persistently numb with poor circulation in my hands and feet.

Besides the four gynecologists I had seen in those two years, I had also gone to naturopaths, osteopaths, acupuncturists, chiropractors, massage therapists, cranial-sacrals, biofeedback practitioners and Chinese herbalists. Not one linked my worsening back problem to the "fibroid" growing steadily on my ovary.

Every time I talked with someone in the medical field about

my symptoms, the conversation came back to my work as being the cause of my back pain. I am an artist. I was specializing at the time in wood sculpture, and was hiking many miles each day collecting wood, carrying it down to my studio and carving it. It was a very physical job, but I always considered it to be healthy. I worked only with hand tools, no chemicals and far away from the hustle and bustle of city life and pollution problems. I was doing what I really enjoyed. Each doctor suggested that I was over stressing my body. In time, my right hand was so painful and numb that I started believing the idea that my work must be the cause. "Carpal tunnel syndrome" was the assumption and soon I was wearing mandatory braces on my wrists and talking with friends about "repetitive motion injury".

If carpal tunnel syndrome is your problem, please take some time to thoroughly research this million dollar industry before you jump into surgery. Order a book by Pete Egoscue called THE EGOSCUE METHOD OF HEALTH THROUGH MOTION. Especially read the section on carpal tunnel syndrome. Do his exercise and if, after a few weeks, things don't improve, then walk in and get your wrist braces and sign up for surgery. But I will make a safe bet that if you do all that Pete Egoscue recommends, your wrists will soon be as good as new.

Ironically, when I was hiking or carving, it was the only time I felt clear-headed and the pain was at its lowest point. I loved walking with my dogs through the thickets of manzanita; it gave me my only peace of mind and body.

It took me quite awhile to prepare myself each day for my long hikes. I would put on my wrist braces, wrap my knees and ankles in ace bandages, and put on a waist brace. What a sight! Sometimes I took two long hikes a day. By then I was convinced there must be something psychologically wrong with me. After all, nothing physical was showing up besides an obvious fibroid tumor and a severe back problem.

It is frightening to see how far from myself I had gone, but all was not lost. Five months before I finally had surgery, I decided to see one more gynecologist who was sixty miles away from my home. He had two offices, one in San Francisco where he did sonograms for hundreds of women each day. His home base was in Mill Valley, a few miles north of San Francisco. He was my age, dapper and very hip with his long ponytail. He ran his office like a fast food drive-thru, with eight examination rooms, each occupied by scantily-clad, shivering women waiting for his appearance and instruction to put their feet in the stirrups. I was one of those women, early on a hot, August day. After giving me a physical exam and a pap smear, he suggested I drive to his office in San Francisco and get another sonogram, my third one in a year and a half.

He was quite sure it was "just a fibroid on your uterus". "But just to be on the safe side, he would do the sonogram." After the exam he suggested I go see his colleague who was a back specialist.

His technician kept redoing my sonagram. She wanted to check something. Her concern combined with "he says this is a fibroid?" made me uneasy. The technician tried to let me leave on a positive note. She said she would confer with the doctor about her concern and I would hear back from him within a week.

Two weeks went by before he finally returned my two phone calls. "Just as I figured," he said smugly, "a very large fibroid tumor on your uterus. Nothing to be concerned about. If you get tired of hauling it around before you start going through menopause, give me a call and we'll talk about zapping that baby out of there. But I bet my career on the fact that as soon as you reach menopause, the fibroid will have left on it's own!"

Before we hung up I mentioned my conversation with his sonogram technician and her questioning the tumor being a fibroid.

"That's why I'm the doctor and she's the technician. We talked about it and she admitted she had made a mistake," he said. I had taped our conversation in case I might need to know some important details. Throughout the following two weeks I went on with what was left of my life - in between the pain. By now I was bleeding every thirteen days for five or six days at a time. It was getting difficult to go to the bathroom and I had to urinate every fifteen minutes. My clothes did not fit well because I had lost so much weight. Eating and loss of appetite were great concerns. I had taken up residence on the living room floor for over a year and sleep occurred in two hour segments under the watchful eye of infomercials.

I thought maybe I should see one more doctor. I would play the tape I made of my conversation with the last gynecologist.

Lost and confused, I was concerned about my thoughts. I had never thought about suicide in my entire life, but now I was thinking about it all day long. My husband and my family were supportive and tried hard to help me. Knowing that killing myself would hurt them tremendously kept me from carrying my thoughts into action.

In one last ditch effort, upon the recommendation of a friend, I made an appointment with a nearby Chinese acupuncturist and herbalist.

While he was treating me for my back, we discussed the fibroid tumor. I asked him if he thought there might be any connection between the two?

"In Western medicine, no. In Eastern medicine, yes," he said in broken English. He continued to tell me that in China "they believe all tumors are bad, even if they are benign. Something is seriously wrong with the body for the immune system to allow a tumor, any tumor, to grow."

I spent many hours thinking about that conversation. Twenty years earlier I had had an ovarian cyst on my right ovary that grew so large that the whole ovary had to be removed. Now, twenty years later, I had ovarian cancer.

During my visit with my Chinese doctor I was still in the dark about the "fibroid", but felt much better just talking with him. He did acupuncture once a week and each week I left his office with seven bags of Chinese herbs to transform daily into a tea. I drank the tea twice a day. Each week I also got a lecture on discipline.

The Chinese doctor told me stories of discipline in China. He said Americans treat their bodies like "spoiled children". He said that spoiling your body until age seven was okay, but after that one needs to learn discipline on a daily basis. Each week I looked forward to hearing a new tale.

I disciplined myself and faithfully drank the tea and did the meditation he prescribed. In just a few weeks my pain was getting tolerable. I was sleeping better and had more strength. The Chinese doctor told me that if the tumor did not show improvement by subsiding within four months, then he would recommend that I return to my gynecologist and have it removed.

During that four month period of drinking the tea, incredible changes were occurring. Some god-awful stuff came out of my body on a daily basis. No longer were my legs swollen and tight. I went for longer periods of time without having to rush to the bathroom. Best of all, I could actually sleep several hours in a row. My back pain was still persistent, but I experienced less of the horrible burning and agonizing pain that comes from severe sciatica.

Within four months of drinking the tea daily and receiving

weekly acupuncture treatments, my "fibroid" actually doubled in size!

It was in the fourth month, just after Christmas, that my Chinese doctor and I made the mutual decision that I now needed to return to my original gynecologist and request surgery.

In early January I was once again reading magazines in another doctor's office. I was given another physical and also a pregnancy test, just in case. The pregnancy test was negative, but the doctor still thought that might be a possibility. She was amazed how large the "fibroid" had gotten since my last visit over six months earlier.

She delayed scheduling surgery until three weeks later because her practice was so hectic. During those three weeks I had ceased taking any more tea. I felt pretty good except the "fibroid" was so large I was again having problems eating, moving my bowels and sleeping. My mind was already geared up for having the fibroid removed. I was looking forward to moving on with my life and feeling better.

The day before my scheduled surgery I went into my gynecologist for pre-op. My husband, David, was with me. Once again I took another pregnancy test. My doctor again was amazed, "how big this thing was"! After my exam she told us that doing surgery the next day was going to be real hard for her. Her schedule was overwhelming! We would have to postpone it!

That was the last straw for me. I lunged out of my chair and if the desk had not been between us, I might have assaulted her. She was very surprised and tried to pacify me by saying "it would just be another couple of weeks - a slight inconvenience".

By then I was on my feet ready to take on anyone who joined in her thinking. I said, "either give me the surgery tomorrow or I'll walk down the street and find someone else who will !" She relented.

I still did not trust her. That night, to insure her participation, David and I plotted to get up at three AM the next morning and go into the emergency room and complain of severe stomach pains. We did that and my doctor was called in to start surgery an hour earlier.

Awakening from surgery is always a bizarre ordeal. For me, still under heavy doses of morphine, it was hallucinatory. David and my family faded in and out of my view. I had not heard the "news" yet but instinctively I wanted to stay wherever I "was." Somewhere music was playing in my head; it was the same "song" being played over and over and it was horrid. Two nurses were discussing the "music" behind me while they adjusted my IV and other devices.

The "music" I heard was agonizing cries from a woman in the next bed. I was in the cancer ward. I was moved to a private room thanks to the understanding and efforts of the nurses. I still did not know they had found cancer during my surgery.

Once situated in my new room, David and my family gathered

around my bed. The time had come to tell me the news. I was still in a drugged state and that helped to soften the blow. David calmly took my hand and with tears in his eyes told me, "Micki, they found the tumor was cancerous. You are fine now. They spent a lot of time looking for more cancer and they believe they got it all."

Wham! The word "cancer" hit me like a two-by-four. Fortunately, a morphine IV was still trickling into my veins. I grabbed David's shirt and pulled him closer to me.

"Are you telling me everything?" I asked gruffly. "You better come clean with me 'cause I want to know it all. So what the hell are we going to do about it?"

David pried loose my hands from his shirt collar. While the James Cagney approach is not healthy for improving one's relationship, I did feel empowered. This was my moment of truth. As groggy as I felt, those twenty-four months of agonizing pain came full circle. Somewhere in my mind, finding out that I had cancer was not news. I already "knew" about it.

David's life also changed at that moment. He would now be thrust into the role of caregiver and for a time, single breadwinner. The abuse he would endure from that point on would not be physical. His pain would come from what I was going through and on occasion, from me.

This is the moment where we shed our skin. Our old life had ended. It would be a long time before his needs would be met and the conversation would shift back to "how's it going with you, David?"

In the many interviews I have done with other people with cancer, it is obvious how frail our relationships become with those who are thrust into the caregiver roles. Their understanding, love, compassion and tolerance are all tested on a daily basis for months, and sometimes years.

Many people have told me how their relationships have changed. We are launched into a "game" of "are you with me or not?" Seldom do you have the time, energy or desire to talk with those close to you and find out what they are really thinking. You may not want to know.

I knew David was "with me". He had been through as much as I had been through in those previous two years. Those earlier months would have been the perfect time for him to have left if he wanted out. I was impossible to live with.

I actually enjoyed the first two days of my hospital stay. Strange to say after learning the cause of all of that pain. I felt a tremendous sense of relief that at least the horror was over and now I could heal. I was being weaned off of the morphine, but I still felt a sense of well-being.

The third day the morphine was gone and the circus of doctors made the rounds to my room several times a day. I was introduced to my oncologist who was my age. This was not a match made in heaven.

My gynecologist came every day, but now that I was lucid, she started every conversation with "I am so sorry I should have...". I spent most of our time together comforting her. She felt badly.

I awakened each day to find the vascular surgeon standing at the foot of my bed. In his dark, pinstriped suit, his white hair and pale skin, he resembled an undertaker and I was startled each time. He checked my six inch wound and reminded me of his name so when I received his bill I would remember who he was and what part he played in this frightful story.

A covey of doctors came through each day - each group asking the same questions, looking at my wound, touching my ankles, scanning my chart. One day I was asked a question that put an end to the mystery of why they were parading so frequently into my room. I had wondered if there was a sign on my door that said "WOMAN WITH ALIEN TUMOR" or what?

Earlier that day the oncologist told me the medical view of my prognosis. I had stage 3B carcinoma, non-differentiated ovarian tumor.

The cancer had spread as two small tumors on my back pelvic wall and also onto all of my reproductive organs and thousands of "seedlings" on the omentum. All of these diseased parts were removed including the culprit itself - my "baby" - an eleven pound cancerous tumor!

After hearing this report, the only thing I could think about was "no wonder I had a back problem!"

The oncologist rattled on about something else, but my mind left the room and scanned the previous two years. It was like I needed to answer those nagging questions that I asked myself each day while in horrible pain. I finally had an answer! Not the answer I really wanted to hear, but it was better then endless wondering.

I smiled and the oncologist stopped in mid sentence. "What's wrong with you?" he asked.

"I'm relieved," I said and smiled some more.

"You're not taking this very seriously," he worried. "Nurse, is she still on a morphine drip?"

The nurse checked my chart to be sure. "No," she said.

Meanwhile, I was moving my back around as best I could while still hooked up to all the paraphernalia. No pain! I lifted my legs individually. No pain! I moved my neck and each arm. The only pain I now felt was where the tumor had lived before it was evicted and the six inch cut from surgery. I smiled some more. The oncologist said he would return later when David was there.

That discovery was short-lived, but a milestone for me. My fear of the cancer was outflanked by this small revelation. My oncologist did not join my celebration. His partypooper attitude was wearing thin.

When the group of doctors, including my oncologist, surrounded my bed later that afternoon, they asked me the question which explained their mysterious behavior.

"In most cases of ovarian cancer, stage 3B, we see tremendous edema in the face, hands, ankles and feet. This wasn't the case for you. Also, when the tumor was exposed and a team of specialists were called in to assist in the surgery, we were surprised to find that your intestines, kidneys and liver were clean and healthy-looking. The cancer had spread but the organs remained healthy. Do you have any idea what you might have done to have such an extremely large tumor and such healthy surroundings?"

It did not take me long to answer. Tales of "discipline" from my Chinese doctor returned. I remembered walking out of his office with seven bags of herbs. I remembered the god-awful "stuff" that came out of my body for many weeks.

"I believe it was the Chinese herbs I drank daily that detoxified my body," I replied. " My Chinese doctor told me that the tumor was growing instead of subsiding because the organs were now able to do their job. The tumor was now retaining the toxins. After four months of watching the tumor grow larger he thought I should have it surgically removed. He said, at that point, there was a chance the tumor could burst. This could be very dangerous and possibly fatal."

A moment of optimism was in their silence. The moment was shattered by one oncologist who snickered and said, "that's the dumbest thing I have ever heard and just not medically possible. The only thing your Chinese doctor understood was the word "malpractice" and he got scared. You have cancer, girlie, and no amount of Chinese herbs is going to cure that; you were just plain lucky. If you want to believe in anything, believe in "karma"; that's what kept you alive."

Anger flushed my face. I was humiliated and underdressed. I pulled the sheet over my body so the group of six men and one woman could no longer view their "specimen". They cackled like chickens and spoke their own language, still discussing their self-imposed mystery.

After that incident I sunk into a depression. Waves of anger, hurt and "why me's?" permeated my room. My internal pain worsened. My intestines that had been inspected so thoroughly during surgery were now rebelling, and spasms riddled my body. The oncologist's belittlement haunted me the rest of the day and through the night.

"...you have cancer, girlie, and no amount of Chinese herbs is going to cure that..." Over and over, his words stung like an angry yellow jacket.

I tried to focus on what my family had put in my room - fun pictures on the wall, cards and flowers and my own art. People came from all over the hospital to see the whimsical animals I had carved. They laughed and said what a wonderful atmosphere it created in my room.

The pain was so bad by this point that the nurse called my doctor and they increased my pain medication. Around midnight

I fell asleep. I woke periodically to the fear of my new realization. I had nightmares of falling into a pit. My vascular surgeon stood over me, dressed in his pinstriped suit, white hair and pale skin. He was kicking dirt on top of me. I was awakened by a nurse to see if I wanted more pain medication. It was five AM. "How fast can you give it to me?" I asked. She laughed and said she would check my vitals and return with the medication.

While waiting for the nurse to return, I saw a pair of small black shoes and tiny legs shuffle through the open door and past the drawn curtain. They looked like shoes my Grandmother had worn, but smaller. I knew it was not the nurse because she wore white shoes.

The small figure hesitated at the edge of the curtain, then slowly peeked around the corner. She was a Mexican woman, very small, just under five feet tall. She was in her late 60's or early 70's. She had beautiful, long, black hair with white streaks. She wore a bright yellow dress with a baby blue crocheted sweater. She looked very friendly but a bit confused when she saw me lying in the bed. She smiled sweetly and looked toward the door, as if she might be in the wrong room.

I remembered hearing people speaking Spanish in the next room the night before. Still smiling, the little lady said "Hi". I returned the salutation and smiled back. I must have looked agonized because she said in broken English, "You...in pain?"

"Yes," I said mournfully, "I'm in terrible pain."

She came closer to the side of the bed. I could smell the faint smell of tacos. She had kind eyes and very white teeth. She wore red lipstick and the creases disappeared when she smiled. She took my large carver's hand, caressed it slowly and said, "I take your pain away."

She raised her other hand above her head and began to chant in Spanish. The tiny hand that held mine was warm and soft. I lay back in silence watching her red lips mouth the Spanish prayer. Her voice rose to such a level, I thought the nurse might come running in. It didn't matter; I just wanted her to stay. I was entranced by her presence.

She stopped chanting as quickly as she had begun. Holding my hand with both of her two tiny hands, she once again told me, "I take your pain away."

Shuffling back toward the curtain, she turned to smile once more. She quietly whispered, "You be okay." Then she was gone.

A minute later the nurse walked through the door and I was disappointed it was not the little lady again.

"I'm sorry I took so long. I got hung up across the hall at the nurses station. You look like you're expecting someone?"

"I thought you might be my little visitor returning...," The nurse cut me off. "What visitor?" she asked.

"The little Mexican woman in the yellow dress. Didn't you see her leave a few minutes ago?"

"I was just across the hall the whole time, and there hasn't been anyone out in the hall for hours. It's five-thirty in the morning."

"She might have gone into the next room. She looked confused like she came into my room by mistake. Last night I heard people speaking Spanish next door so that's where she probably went."

The nurse started taking my pulse. "There was a young Mexican man in the next room, but I"m sorry to say he died yesterday. He didn't have any visitors while he was here. We felt badly for him. Now the room is empty. I think you have lost track of time because of the pain medication. Sometimes hallucinations are one of the side effects."

The nurse gave me my pain medication, turned off the light and pulled the curtain across the door. I was troubled by the idea that this beautiful, gentle lady was just a figment of my drug-induced mind. How could this be? I thought I even smelled her. My hand still lingered with her warmth. I felt her baby blue crocheted sweater brush my skin. Those red lips entranced me with loud chanting. I watched the curtain door for as long as I could before the medication kicked in and I could no longer remain awake.

It was nine AM before I awoke from my deep and restful sleep. David was sitting by my bed reading the newspaper. The room was bright and filled with early February sunlight. I told David I felt like walking the halls. He called the nurse so I could move the portable IV. Swinging my legs to the side of the bed, David remarked how easy I was able to do that maneuver. I was amazed also. I stood up. No pain, just a slight spasm in my intestines.

Walking the halls, I felt better than I had for the last two years. When we were back in the room I told David about the "little lady". I mentioned my disappointment that it was probably the medication. I could still see her sweet face clearly, hear her chant and smell her clothes. It did not seem possible that she was an illusion.

That day in the hospital was my best day. Without pain I was able to get off the medication and be unhooked from all apparatus. It was Sunday and the entourage of doctors were nowhere to be seen. My gynecologist called and said if I improved as much in the next 24 hours as the last day that I could possibly go home on Monday.

That night I felt strong and ... fearless. Yes, that was it. That is what was missing, the fear. I no longer cowered when the cancer was brought up. I focused on what I was going to do when I got home: David, my art, my family - my healing.

Monday morning I was told I could leave the hospital around noon. I had to meet with my oncologist to discuss "his plans for my future."

Sitting at the end of my bed, stern-faced and serious, my oncologist proceeded to tell David and me how I would be spending the next year and a half of my life.

"Because you had a non-differentiated tumor that had spread we must do a year, maybe longer, of chemotherapy. We'll start out with two common chemotherapy drugs and if, after six months, you're still not out of the woods, then we'll switch to two others. We'll schedule the chemotherapy treatments every 28 days. We've scheduled a port-a-cath to be put in your chest area in a minor surgical procedure for next week. The "port" allows the chemotherapy to go directly into the heart and into the bloodstream faster and more efficiently than an IV in the vein.

A week later we will start the treatments. We will also need to get a blood test from you before the chemotherapy to check your CA-125. (A tumor marker test for Ovarian cancer. Normal range is 0 to 35) Your CA-125 right after surgery was 2400, which is high and indicated to us that your cancer cells are proliferating. I will have you come to my office prior to the treatment so we can discuss further any questions you both may have after thinking about this for a few days." Then he left the room. David and I felt tense and anxious.

I was happy to get to the car where our three dogs were waiting for us. They squeaked with glee, shaking their butts and tails back and forth, so happy to see me. As I held one of my dogs in my arms on the drive home I thought of the "little lady". I was torn between two worlds. One, where I felt comfortable and unafraid - the other cold, confusing and separate from myself.

Whether the "little lady" was an illusion or not, "seeing" her made a difference in my life. When she said, "I will take your pain away," I thought she was talking about my physical pain. That was gone. So was my fear and the paralyzing feeling I had experienced since the words "you have cancer" entered my mind.

At home I sat in different chairs I had not sat in for almost two years, because of the sciatica. I was able to drive again, walk without a cane and without braces. Gone were the "carpal tunnel syndrome," the back pain, the sciatic pain, the headaches, the insomnia, the metallic taste in my mouth. They were all gone. I might have come home with the "proliferating cancer cells" but that was okay. I was home, I was alive and I had met a beautiful, magical, "little lady".

Two weeks after my surgery, with a "port" now surgically implanted in my chest, I marched in like a good soldier and reported for chemotherapy. Sitting in the lounge chair, while going through the treatment, I recalled a conversation I had the week before with my oncologist.

"Should I take any special precautions while I'm going through this treatment?" I asked.

"Try to stay away from very sick people," was his reply.

I looked around the "chemotherapy room," the only people

in the room were sick! Very sick and dying people!

The chemotherapy treatment was uneventful until the next day and throughout the following week when the typical nausea reared its ugly head. Terrifying headaches started in my eyes and moved over my entire head and made the ground shake beneath me. For several days I experienced those horrible symptoms.

A week later my hair vacated the premises. My body was one toxic waste dump and my hair would have no part of it ! It fell out.

Recuperating from the treatment, I had some time to read and talk with friends. I was told about a medical center in San Diego where they work on boosting your immune system to hold off the cancer. In California (and most other States) the only legal method of treating cancer is with surgery, chemotherapy or radiation. No one else can say they are treating cancer or the facility will be closed by the Food and Drug Administration.

I told my oncologist I was considering the Livingston Medical Center in San Diego for their two week immune boosting program. He had nothing good to say about the Center. He called them "charlatans" and expressed his fear of their inhumane way of treating dying people.

He then went into how much money Livingston charged patients when I interrupted and said, "Excuse me, are your services free? Tell me, how much does chemotherapy cost?" He interrupted with "They have no data down there at that center...".

I rudely cross-fired, "SHOW ME YOUR DATA!"

He went off on another subject. "If you don't do chemotherapy for at least one year you won't be celebrating the next New Year." I brought him back to the "data" issue. Eventually he relented and had his secretary bring in data of women who had the same stage ovarian cancer as I did, and who had followed his recommendation of one year or more of chemotherapy.

When I read it I was more flabbergasted than I expected to be - they had all died within two years! I stood up and dropped the "data" on the floor like it was contagious. "Are you kidding me?" I said with great calm, "I'd have a better chance in Las Vegas betting all on the red!"

Our argument went on but it was pointless. If I was "dying" why was I arguing limitations with a pompous medical doctor?

Two weeks later I was on a flight to San Diego.

At the Livingston Medical Center in San Diego, I walked in the first morning at 7:30 AM and deposited several vials of blood to their lab. I also left a urine and stool sample, and a lock of my hair. They also pricked blood from my finger to do a darkfield microscope reading.

After all the paperwork was completed, I was sent to their

cafeteria to eat breakfast made by their resident chef.

That first day I kept busy getting acquainted with the staff and the eight other people who were going through the program with me. Other people mingled and waltzed in and out for two-day visits while they received annual checkups.

They were the walking "data" my oncologist insisted that Livingston did not have. I'll take that kind of "data" any day. People were from every part of the country. They had every conceivable cancer and they were still around to talk about it five, ten, fifteen years later.

The second day I was given a schedule of how my time would be filled for the following two weeks. I met my doctor for the first time that afternoon. He had already conferred with the nutritionist over my blood report.

When I walked in the door for the first time, I got the sense that I was embraced by people who were interested in me individually. They made every effort to move me through the process quickly, but pleasantly. They worked hard to find out as soon as possible what my body needed to get my immune system functioning to as near normal as possible.

There were two other women going through the program with me who also had ovarian cancer. One was in her late sixties, the other was on her first recurrence after eight years. She was now 32. My cancer, in medical terms, was more advanced then theirs, yet I was healthier then either of them. The program designed for me was streamlined and less costly in comparison. By the second week my blood work had surpassed the normal expected criteria.

At breakfast or lunch we would talk candidly about our individual experiences with cancer, doctors, hospitals and our families. What a treat not to worry about other people feeling queasy about cancer.

I thrived at the Livingston Center, but some people did not. A couple who started the program with me came from Michigan with their three young children. Livingston was the last hope for the husband who had liver cancer. He was 35 years old; his wife was the same age. Just six months earlier the cancer was discovered in an exam for pain in his back. He was assaulted with heavy doses of twice weekly chemotherapy and his tumor was considered inoperable.

After four months of this barrage on his body, the doctors gave up and told him and his wife to get their affairs in order. When his wife told his doctors they would be coming to the Livingston Center, they suggested he should "be fitted for a coffin upon his arrival".

They sold possessions at home so they could make the trip. Their three children came with them because they did not want to be separated and Kevin was being realistic. With no encouragement from anyone in their families they journeyed to San Diego. Kevin was in extreme pain. His body was emaciated except for the swollen stomach area which housed the tumor. He looked like he was nine months pregnant.

My heart broke when I met this family. In cancer, there is no such thing as "fair play".

The first four days Kevin joined us at the cafeteria. He and his wife had small glimmers of hope, but his body was reacting to the surge of nutrition and vaccines, which were only temporary. The days that followed were unrelenting for all of us. Our small victories were short- lived when we heard the reports on Kevin.

He made a decision that he would not die in San Diego because of the expense and hassle for his wife and children. He was carried to the ambulance that took him to their flight back home. He would have to sit up in a seat for the five hour return flight to Michigan. It must have been horrendous and he was very brave. These would be his last few hours alive, and he was aware of that. Kevin kept his promise and died two hours after arriving home.

There are many stories like Kevin's at the Livingston Center but more common are the stories like mine.

No longer am I surviving. I passed surviving many moons ago. My magic word is THRIVING!

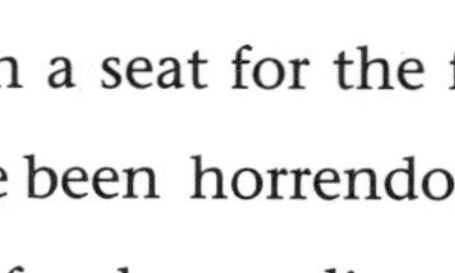

Cancer takes tremendous effort and time to overtake it. After the Livingston program I kept up their regime, but also did everything and "the kitchen sink" to stay well. The payoff was a total return to work within four months after surgery and diagnosis. I was back to hand-carving whimsical and humorous animals and hiking the hills with David and my beloved dogs and cats.

My name was put on a list by the Cancer Control Society in Los Angeles, California, as a patient who did non-toxic therapy. The calls started coming in several times a week the first year, and almost daily after that. Are more people getting cancer? The statistics now are 1 in 3 people will get some form of cancer. I believe more people are questioning the present "treatments" and are no longer marching in to report for chemotherapy or radiation as they did in the last thirty years. The "walking data" does not lie.

In the following chapters are the 15 decisions I have compiled through my conversations with the hundreds of people who are talking loudly. They want alternative methods of healing.

I now incorporate my art with public speaking, and talk on ART AND HEALING. People are angry about their medical treatments, their HMO's and the fact that doctors protect each other, and take too little time to humanize Western medicine.

There is a "spring" after the "winter" of cancer. Besides fate and destiny, it takes hard work and tremendous belief in what you are doing. You must design a treatment that works for you, and you alone.

DECIDE within the first fifteen minutes if you want to overcome this disease or not. This seems obvious, but it is rarely considered until the shock wears off. You must make this a priority. It is beneficial for the mind to focus immediately on healing.

CHAPTER THREE

When someone calls me for information on non-toxic approaches to cancer treatments I ask, "How did you react when you first heard the news about your diagnosis with cancer?" "How did you handle it?"

I am intrigued by their answers. Some are simple and to the point. "I fainted." "I dropped to my knees." "My heart started to race."

Others are more graphic. "I left the room crying and got in my car and drove crazy for 10 miles before I became aware of what I was doing." "My husband and I broke every dish in the kitchen and felt overwhelmed." Still others quietly have said, "I asked, Why me?"

News of hearing, "You have cancer" can devastate the most controlled individual. Very few of us are prepared for this event. It is easy to believe it will happen to someone else but, "to me?" is devastating.

Many people, like myself, pride themselves in believing they have done everything possible to keep from getting this insidious disease. We have eaten the fruits and vegetables we are told will save us from harm. We have exercised to the point of obsession. We have lived in an environment that is supposed to be healthy.

Then there are the "I'm not going to worry about it" people. Who eat junk food, do not take vitamins, and stress themselves out.

There are the people who are the most sweet and lovable individuals you could ever meet, alongside the folks who are the meanest and most cantankerous. I have talked with them all. They all had one thing in common - they heard someone tell them those three unforgettable words: "You have cancer."

Hearing those words sends shockwaves through every part of your body, not only physically. I have learned that what is going on in the mind in that moment is critical to initiate healing. I have been told that many people "take a short trip" when they first hear they have cancer. Where do they go? Their minds "visit" everyone they can recall who they ever knew had cancer. It's like searching for a file in your brain. The file heading is "CANCER". It's opened up and out flow memories of people one has known who were "struck down" by this disease. Few people actually knew more than five people who were still living normal lives after having cancer, or who were living at all. They make that comparison and WHAM, "You're a goner," flashes foremost in their heads.

We recall the emaciated bodies we have seen from our experience with relatives and friends suffering and dying from cancer. Few people I talked with had healthy thoughts of anyone they knew with this disease.

I made notes of people that said very little about their initial reaction to the devastating news. They either did not recall much about the event, or it had not been something they focused on. How is that possible? Most often, something beyond their control happened at the same time.

Recalled months later, they seemed to fare better in their healing journey. I saw a pattern. What was the pattern? I can best relay it with one of my favorite stories of a woman named Kathy, who three years later, believes her initial response was a big part of her healing.

When Kathy called me, she had been diagnosed two months earlier. She had just had her surgery. She was told she had stage 3C ovarian cancer. When I asked her, "what was your reaction upon first hearing the news?" Her answer was, "I don't really remember because I fainted."

"What happened when you woke up ?" I asked.

She snickered and replied, "I still don't remember, probably because of the fire."

"What fire?" My curiosity was burning.

"Well, it was very strange. I had just gotten home from work. I was cooking pork chops on the stove when I saw the red light flashing on my answering machine. I listened to the messages and one was from my gynecologist whom I had seen earlier in the week. He was giving me the results of a sonogram and blood test I had taken. He sounded deadpanned at first, so I listened intently, but expected nothing unusual. Very casually he said the words, "...and so it looks like you have an advanced stage of cancer but we will know more when we open you up..." the next thing I know, I was getting oxygen by a paramedic out on the front lawn of my townhouse."

"Apparently when I fainted, the pork chops burned and started the kitchen on fire. My neighbors heard the smoke alarm and saw the smoke. They ran in and pulled me out of the house. Soon the fire department and paramedics were there. My kitchen was gutted and there was a lot of smoke damage."

"What did you do about the news of the cancer?" I was intrigued.

"Nothing. At least for a month I did nothing. I didn't even get back to my doctor for three weeks, and he never bothered to call me back. I was displaced from my house and moved in with friends for at least a month. I had enough to do trying to get my house back in shape. Dealing with the insurance company was a nightmare, and cleaning up the smoke damage was unbelievable! It was after I moved back into the house when I finally could focus on the cancer surgery. By then, it was just something else I had to deal with... I knew it was important but it seemed anticlimactic!"

Kathy did have surgery and one cycle of chemotherapy. She was scheduled to do a second cycle of chemotherapy when the "cosmos intervened" once again. Driving to her treatment with a friend, they were sideswiped by a drunk-driver and pushed off the road. They were unhurt but the car had to be towed. Kathy missed her appointment and never returned. She thought this vehicular intervention was a "sign".

She called me to find out about my experience in non-toxic cancer treatments. In the end, she chose an alternative treatment. With no more "cosmic interferences", she is doing very well at this writing.

Most stories do not have the drama of Kathy's. Her mind reached overload and spared her from the bad news. Kathy thought, "What else can happen?" She views it as a fortunate break. Being sideswiped and pushed off the road by a drunk-driver, she even considers a blessing.

Fainting saved Kathy from herself, but what about the rest of those fortunate few? Like Keith.

Keith's fate had a manmade twist to it. For several months Keith felt pretty lousy. He went in for a checkup, did a full blood panel and got the "works". After all was said and done, he was told, everything "looked great and his blood work looked like a twenty year old." Keith went about his business, but still felt lousy two months later.

This time he decided to give himself a treat. He took a month off from work and went to a well-known spa in Europe. He thought he needed some R&R.

Keith was pampered and relaxed at the spa. He exercised daily, meditated, drank lots of juices and ate only organic foods. No telephones, no TV, none of the invasive electronics he lived with at home. Keith was a happy camper.

After three weeks at the spa, Keith traveled through Europe for another two weeks before heading home. After settling in at home, Keith received a phone call from the first doctor who did his blood test before he left for Europe. His doctor requested that Keith come to his office. "It was urgent that they talk."

At his doctor's office, Keith sat in dead silence. His doctor relayed the mixup of Keith's files with that of another patient taking the same blood test in the hospital on the same day as Keith. That other patient was a twenty year old man who was taking a required physical for a new job. Keith's blood work was put in the other patient's file and vice versa. No wonder Keith's blood looked like that of a "twenty year old". Keith was 53 years old.

There was bad news; Keith had a rare form of Leukemia. The mixup was discovered when the other patient was told he had Leukemia. After giving the other patient several new blood tests and finding them negative, the hospital investigated. They researched other patients who were tested on the same day and discovered the error.

Keith was devastated by the news. He took another blood panel. His blood work still showed signs of Leukemia, but there was an extreme difference from the original blood work a few months earlier! His doctor was amazed, and suggested that Keith hold off any standard treatment for Leukemia and wait another month for more testing.

Keith called me to talk about recommendations for alternative treatment centers here in the United States. He had used most of his vacation time, but had sick leave saved. He also had spent his budget on the European trip, so he needed to stay closer to home.

Keith chose a doctor closer to home. He was given a treatment similar to what he experienced at the European spa. He called me back two months later to report that his Leukemia was in remission.

Bernie had just turned eighteen when his tongue discovered a lump on the roof of his mouth. He mentioned it to his parents. They set him up with an appointment with a doctor at their HMO. A biopsy was taken, and the tumor was lasered and removed in a surgical procedure in the hospital. The doctor said the biopsy was negative, but he felt it needed another look. The biopsy was sent to another lab where the results took several weeks. Bernie healed quickly and went about his busy summer.

Several months later, Bernie's father, who shares the same first and last name, went to the same hospital for an examination. His doctor looked at his file and asked how he was feeling since the cancer?

Confused by the doctor's comment, Bernie Senior said he

"didn't have cancer." The doctor said that his chart showed he had surgery six months earlier and the result of the biopsy revealed carcinoma cancer. The confusion disclosed the mixup with the charts of Bernie Junior and Bernie Senior.

When informed about the confusion, Bernie Junior heard for the first time that the tumor on his cleft palate had been carcinoma. The doctor who performed the surgical procedure spoke with a heavy accent. The combination of the accent, along with Bernie executing his right to his independence at age eighteen, led to the confusion. Bernie went in for a checkup after the surgery without anyone present. The doctor must have said the words "carcinoma cancer" but Bernie never heard it. He told his mother, he had a hard time understanding the doctor, but that everything was fine.

By the time the discovery was made, the original doctor had left that hospital. Bernie's file had been put in with his father's file. Bernie received no medical treatment for his cancer. The second doctor advised him that the type of cancer he had served as no hazard to his health. He is healthy today.

For a time, these three people were spared the news of their disease, and fortunately it worked out to their benefit. For many people, including myself, a misdiagnosis or no diagnosis could have been fatal.

I am intrigued by those first fifteen minutes of truth, when someone is told about their cancer. Without the bungling of others to sabotage the impending news, is it possible to create our own Mr. Magoo attitude when first hearing the news?

A woman nicknamed "Cricket" called me one gray winter day, to talk about her alternative choices for healing and to tell me what took place when she was told she had Stage 3 ovarian cancer.

In the previous five years, she had run four marathons and considered herself to be quite fit and healthy. The last marathon she doubled up in pain many times throughout the race, but finished in the top twenty. Heavy bleeding occurred, and Cricket knew something was out of sorts. She went to her gynecologist a week later and had a physical exam, a blood test, and a sonogram. Cricket was given an appointment to review the sonogram three days later.

On her way, Cricket pulled her car over to the side of the road and decided to "make a deal with herself".

"What sort of deal did you make?" I asked.

"The deal was this: if I was okay, I would give up running marathons and settle down and focus on making a better living. Or if I wasn't okay, then I would continue to run marathons until I dropped dead, shake my life up more and focus on living better!"

Cricket promised herself that whatever she was told that she could handle it and concentrate on healing. She planned to run in the next scheduled marathon in Hawaii in six months.

Sitting across from her gynecologist, Cricket heard the words, "You have an ovarian tumor. Your blood test reveals that it is cancerous."

"Did your "deal" work out the way you planned?" I desperately wanted to know.

"Yes!" Cricket said emphatically. "I felt empowered! As disciplined as I was in training for marathons, I used that same discipline with my mind. When I heard my gynecologist say those words, 'You have cancer' I took several long deep breaths and kept my cool."

Cricket had surgery soon afterward and a hysterectomy. She went to the Simonton Cancer Center in Santa Barbara and pursued mind techniques and healthy living. She made her goal of running the marathon in Hawaii, and has run three other marathons since our original conversation.

Cricket was accustomed to discipline. I have talked with other people who never expected such devastating news, who then made the instant decision to overcome their "dis-ease" and concentrate on healing. That first fifteen minutes is crucial, but it is never too late to start focusing on healing. If you are reading this book 3, 6, or even 12 months after your diagnosis, you can still make a healing decision.

At this moment of truth, you must learn to empower yourself, and be focused on how you are going to heal.

I was fortunate. I had three days of morphine to dope up my mind. When I was told the news, David said it took three times for me to understand. It was a "lost file". It was three days before I could clearly digest the information.

I do not advocate getting doped up before you sit down with your doctor and prepare for the bad news, or hoping that the cosmos intervenes. I believe we can do better.

We can DECIDE how we are going to filter the news, even if that decision is made on the spot.

Many of us have lost spontaneity in our lives. When we were children we did not hesitate to make a decision. As grownups, we no longer feel good or sure of an instant decision. We have so much to think about. We need to weigh the facts, to consider all of the ramifications. We have learned that instant decisions can be costly and unplanned.

When you have a life-threatening "dis-ease", all of that "grownup stuff" disappears anyway, or it should. Your life is at stake. DECIDING to save yourself is a very good start. Make this your priority!

Pay attention to your BREATHING. Take long, slow, deep breaths. Calm yourself as much as possible - do not allow this news to overwhelm you!

CHAPTER FOUR

Most of us do not realize the destruction that takes place in the body when we constrict our natural breathing pattern. By the time we have made it to our early twenties, we have "relearned" how to breathe. Or more correctly, how "not" to breathe.

Breathing is an odd occurrence. The healthy person does it without any effort. It is only when our breathing is interrupted or threatened that we consciously give it any thought.

Twenty minutes without oxygen and we are considered brain dead. Soon after, the rest of the body conforms, ending our life.

By the time a person is diagnosed with cancer, their oxygen depletion has already developed, subtlety. When I asked if someone could remember if they had felt shortness of breath or lack of energy prior to their diagnosis of cancer, they all responded, "Yes!"Looking back on my own experience, I remember having to expend more energy to do things I had normally done earlier with ease. Breathing, during that year prior to my surgery, was an issue that came up many times in my conversations. Because of pollution, age, lack of sleep, it never made an impression on me.

By the time we have reached our early twenties our normal intake of oxygen has been significantly reduced . Where does all of that energy come from in children? If they are normal, they are using 100% of their oxygen intake. When they have reached their teens, they have slowly started their decline of efficient oxygen metabolization.

Each one of us learns how "not" to breathe during those formative years. Depending on our personal lives, our relationships, our role models - how we act or react to our experiences - all of this training adds up to the final quotient. We have retaught ourselves how to breathe.

Have you continually had experiences in your life that upset your stomach? Have you experienced daily fear or disappointment? The parade of emotions is endless. The mere experiencing of these emotions will not give you cancer. What will increase your chances of getting cancer is your continued lack of oxygen while you deal with the stresses of life.

When "bad news" is a constant in your life and you do not learn how to rid yourself of your reaction to that news, you have also "forgotten" to breathe. Cancer cells thrive in poorly oxygenated systems.

Twelve of five hundred people I interviewed, who had been diagnosed with cancer, were serious marathon runners. Twenty-two were serious bicyclists. These two sports are known for increased oxygen intake.

Take this one step further and the interviews indicate that most of these thirty-four people said they had significant "breathing" problems. Sports increased their oxygen intake, but they also depleted their oxygen absorption in their daily struggles.

The moments they were diagnosed with cancer were probably

moments of fear. Most people don't remember if they were breathing or not, but they do remember feeling short of breath, feeling faint and lightheaded.

Only two people remembered how they controlled their breathing during that crucial moment. One person was Cricket who struck a deal with herself and followed through by taking long, slow, deep breaths.

The other person was Elaine. She launched into a chant the minute the words came out of her doctor's mouth. Elaine said her doctor was startled. She thought it was a good way to set the stage for their continued relationship. Whenever he discussed his negative opinion, she started chanting. He stopped giving her his opinion.

Elaine continues to chant daily, and feels it gives her the calming influences she needs. I agree with Elaine. I too chant on a regular basis.

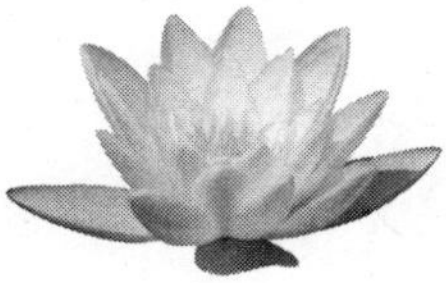

The influence of cancer is widespread. Be prepared for that person who tells you, "my aunt or uncle died of the same cancer."

Or you turn on the TV or radio just in time to hear the latest statistics on how many people are dying from cancer. Take several long, slow, deep breaths to help remove you from those frightening moments. Prayer is also powerful.

Throughout the day, pay close attention to your breathing. See how you feel when you're in a good mood. Notice the difference in your breathing when something upsets you or you feel lousy. Get in the habit of taking deep breaths once an hour. Learn how to use this powerful and natural tool, and you will seldom be overwhelmed by "bad news". Control your breathing during those "fight or flight" moments, for it is a dynamic tool in your healing experience. It's free, it's natural and it has worked magic for many people. Don't forget to use it.

The words "Cancer" and "AIDS" have a profound and powerful effect on our society. Turn that around. Replace your thinking with words that propel you to action. You will need to call on your PERSONAL POWER often. Learn to use it.

CHAPTER FIVE

When people call me about Cancer, the subject always comes up about the impact of the words "Cancer" and "AIDS". It is not surprising the effect these words have on each one of us. I talk with some people who are very successful. They run their own businesses and have lots of money in the bank . Yet when they hear the word "Cancer", they cower like a frightened dog.

Paralyzed from fear, they tell me they can no longer function. For the first time in their lives, they feel weak and helpless.

Through these conversations, I am reminded of the spirit that dwells within each of us. Most of us don't know the mighty force that we have inherited - that glorious gift called PERSONAL POWER!

No matter how despondent or despairing a person becomes, there is always a spark of personal power to revitalize. Many times I have been moved to tears hearing the stories of those who found their strength of character before they withered away. I have been moved by those who could not drag themselves from the terrifying pit created by their own fears. Each still had a spark of personal power. Waiting to be called upon, that power is always there. It only dies when we die.

I received a call from a woman named Caroline. At first I thought it was a business call until somewhere in the conversation she glossed over the word CANCER. I thought I heard her say she had "Breast cancer", but her tone was like listening to a report.

After a few minutes, I interrupted and blatantly asked, "Why are you calling me?"

"I have breast cancer and I've been told you can give me some suggestions for possible alternative treatment centers? I'm pursuing conventional medicine treatments, but I would like to complement those treatments with some alternative methods. Here is my fax number. Please fax all of your information to me and my secretary will be in touch if I have any more questions. Thank you very much." Click. She hung up.

As devoted as I am to helping people, I do have my limits. I do not get paid for talking with people on the telephone or faxing them "all of my information". Caroline tapped my limits of compassion. I threw away her fax number and went about my business.

Three days later she left me a message and reminded me of the fax. She said she would appreciate me writing a letter of recommendation about the Livingston Medical Center so she can give that to her insurance company.

Stubbornly, I held off any correspondence until I heard from her personally. The following week she did call me. This time she sounded sheepish.

Caroline was all business, even with her own disease. She asked about my experience at the Livingston Center. Would she have to actually stay there *two weeks* ? Then she rattled on about how many Board of Directors she was on, her time schedule, her daughter's upcoming wedding. She saw no way that she could do the vaccines that were part of the Livingston program. With all of the traveling she and her husband did, it would be very difficult to move the vaccines through Customs.

The Livingston diet would also create havoc in her life. Three times a year, she and her husband went to their chateau in the South of France. The thought of giving up wine was out of the question.

I sat quietly feeling like Alice in Wonderland listening to the March Hare.

Caroline called me twice after our initial conversation. Each time I detected a frightened rabbit in executive armor. In our conversations she rarely, if at all, said the word "Cancer". When she did say it, I was convinced she was talking about a product from her company. I had images of her constantly checking her watch and babbling, "I'm late. I'm late. For a very important date."

In our last conversation, Caroline said she would consider her possibilities and when she had time she would pursue some alternative direction.

A year later, I answered the telephone to a weak voice on the other end. Unbelievably, it was Caroline. She talked very soft and slowly, and I could feel her pain in her voice.

We talked about her experiences of the last year. She said she did nothing to heal herself except the chemotherapy. She ate what she always ate, worked long hours, raced around the world in their private jet, and drank lots of wine in the South of France.

"Sounds like you've been having a great time," I said with a twinge of envy.

"I guess someone would think that," Caroline said softly. "But with very little time left, I must tell you, I have been scared to death. I thought I could run faster than the cancer. I've been successful at everything else."

I couldn't believe the change. Caroline was in total despair. She knew her life was nearing the end. She said the cancer had spread throughout her body. I asked her why she didn't take better care of herself.

"All I could focus on was the word, CANCER. I never could get past it. It paralyzed me. Even when I looked like I was having a good time, inside my mind I tossed that word around like a tennis ball. Cancer meant failure to me. I heard conversations of people talking about someone who had cancer. They talked in low and hushed tones, shaking their heads in pity. I could never tell anyone I was one of those pitiful people."

"Is there a reason that you're calling me back?" I asked.

"No" she said tearfully. "Well yes... I wanted to see if you were still alive. I need to tell you... I, uh, I was very envious of you when we first talked. I wanted what you have. I didn't know what that was right away, but I figured it out a few months later."

"What was that?" I asked, burning with curiosity.

"You seem unstoppable. You have... personal power. I thought I had that, but it was only in the area of money. When it came to personal strength, I found myself overcome by fear. Where did you get your strength?" Caroline paused.

"From people and experiences in my life," I said, "but mainly from people like yourself who don't know it, but your personal power has come alive."

"I do know it," she said proudly, "I recognized it the day I took my watch off! On my last visit to France, I read a poem in the stall of a cafe bathroom. Translated from French, it goes like this: "My life is but a little thing; but it is - MY LIFE!"

Caroline's life ended one month later. She was 48 years old.

Every person in this world is capable of setting their own course, even when that course is healing from cancer. We are built to overcome the difficulties we encounter. We are free to drift or progress as we choose. Personal power is the inward force that drives each one of us. It is something more than intelligence, because it makes one use their intelligence in the right way. It is something more than character, for it creates character. It is something more than personality, for personality is but an expression of one's mind.

It is more than all these things. It gives one the eye to see beauty, the mind to appreciate life in its fullness, and the strength to grasp what one needs to overcome the hand they were dealt.

Even in times of despair, personal power lies dormant within you, waiting and able to turn despair into hope.

I was fortunate to have a role model thirty years ago who taught me, very simply, that personal power exists in all of us, at any time. My role model was my mother. While in her forties she discovered a lump in her breast. It was cancerous. At that time the only course of action was a radical mastectomy. After she healed from surgery she returned to her doctor and asked him what she should do next. "You have five children, don't you?" My mother nodded, "Yes." "Then go home and take care of them, you'll be fine" he said.

She did go home and took care of her children. She also ran in a 10K race soon after her surgery. It wasn't very easy at that time. People didn't talk about cancer at all. There were no support groups and people were quite suspicious of possibly "catching" cancer. There was no reconstructive surgery for breast cancer, as there is today.

My mother, Jean, gathered her personal power and went on with her life. She was a housewife. Her theory on the success of living was simple. There can be no success for living without strength of character! Her strength came from her spiritual beliefs, her family - but also, from within herself.

No one can foster your personal power, not your family, your doctor, your care giver - only you. It is yours alone. You are the only one who can develop it; you alone can use it.

Many times, I am sure my mother felt alone and frightened, even with her large family around. Instead of allowing herself to be terrified by her difficulties and fears, she fixed her thoughts on successfully living. A year or two after my mother's breast cancer surgery, Shirley Temple Black and Happy Rockefeller both developed breast cancer. The path got a little easier for women after these two public individuals shared their experience with the world. It also opened up the world of chemical therapy - chemotherapy and radiation soon became the "popular" way of treatment.

That "path" was well-worn already by thousands of other women who dealt with their cancer quietly, but forcefully. A lot of them are still around and still vital and healthy, including my mother.

There is no doubt that the word cancer has a frightening history, but we can avail ourselves to the experience of others. We can open ourselves not only to their knowledge, but more importantly, to their wisdom.

Fix your thoughts on successfully living and on that inward force, your PERSONAL POWER !

Do not ask, "How long do I have?". Your doctor can only give you a scientific generalization. You are a unique individual with a unique immune system.

CHAPTER SIX

Sadly, when many people I have interviewed reached the point of discussing their prognosis with their oncologist, they became paralyzed with fear. Earlier with their cancer, they did well with controlling their fear. They were busy getting adjusted to their new life or they were convalescing from recent surgery. Some had gone through the recommended one to two years of chemotherapy. They anxiously awaited the final results of their dedication toward that treatment, only to hear that their cancer is "aggressive" and there is no cure. The patient is baited and they ask the unforgiving question, "How long do I have?"

Most of the time, the answer is never what they wanted or expected to hear. With people I interview, this question, "How long do I have?" brings out the most contempt. Though many believed in their doctors and freely asked the question, the finality angered them.

Michael was a 48 year old psychotherapist with an inoperable brain tumor. He was furious when his doctor told him there was no more hope and that he should go home and get his affairs in order. I asked him what he said to his doctor after he was told he had six months to live?

"After five minutes of expletives, I asked him, 'Who do you think you are telling me something like that?' His doctor said, 'It's not a matter of who I think I am, it's scientific data. A mechanic can determine by looking at your brake pads how long before your brakes will fail. Through my education and my experience, I can come close to the same determination. It would take an absolute miracle for you to survive any longer than six months with this brain tumor.' By then I was busting mad! I wanted to break every bone in this guy's body! Imagine being compared to your automobile's brake pads! My gosh, I could come up with a better example than that! But I knew getting angrier at him wouldn't solve anything. I just told him to clear his computer for some fresh, new data - ME ! I told him he was limited by his education and somewhere along the way he stopped learning. He needed to get out of his office, the hospital, his computer and start opening his mind to possibilities not absolutes!"

Michael continued for five minutes. "All of my life I believed in medical science. There were three doctors in my immediate family. For the first time I saw the dishonesty of this profession. Patting themselves on the back for their many years of formal education, doctors are convinced they have learned it all. Instead, their learning ended when they got their degree. No one, I repeat, NO ONE can honestly say how long someone has to live. If they do, and the person believes them, then I am convinced that the doctor is like someone who practices voodoo. They're sticking 'needles' in someone's mind and that's what is killing the person!"

Michael was obviously upset, but his "fire" must have paid off. While writing this book, two and a half years after our last conversation, Michael called me. It was great to hear from him. After our first conversation, his tumor disappeared for over a year. Michael went down to the Bahamas to Dr. Lawrence Burton's Clinic and stayed on their program for two years. The tumor showed up again in a CT scan a year later. Michael still has control over the tumor at present and is working and maintaining his lifestyle.

Through these interviews, I have learned how listening to people and being guided by them exclusively, binds us by the limits of their minds. That includes doctors, anyone in the medical profession, or those in alternative medicine. We are all limited by our "education", no matter how extensive. Education is useless when understanding a person's inner thoughts and the capacity of their mind. When we find out we have cancer, we know our own thoughts and become acquainted with the capacity of our minds. I have learned that the limit of one's powers is the limit of one's mind, and it expands proportionately through use.

I am reminded of a demure, young woman who called me one day from the Midwest. Her name was Marlene and she was crying uncontrollably. Marlene was 28 years old, a single mother of two children, and desperate. Following surgery her sister had just dropped her off at her home after her third visit to her oncologist. Marlene had ovarian cancer, stage 3. Her tumor was removed and the cancer had not metastasized. Her biggest concern was her children, ages three and eight.

"What is your concern for them?" I asked.

"I've only got a few months to live and I have to figure out who will take them and love them."

"Who told you that you only have a few months to live?" I acted surprised.

"I just came from my oncologist's office and he said with chemotherapy I would probably live up to two years, and without it, probably only four or five months. I don't have insurance so I'm sunk."

I could feel the hair on the back of my neck bristle from anger. This was the moment that I expected to meet one day. The moment when I would witness the collision of someone's American Dream with the reality of a disease. Married at eighteen, she dropped out of high school, Marlene said her marriage lasted six years. Her husband had not been seen or heard from for over two years. She worked as a waitress at a local restaurant. No insurance for her or her children, and now, she ended up with cancer. Her surgery was covered by the county, but her oncologist refused to take county payments and she was paying $95 for each visit. He offered her no hope past two years, even though her cancer was limited to the tumor that was removed.

It took every ounce of restraint to control my anger. I wanted to show her my empathy, not my temper.

"How old do you think this oncologist-with-an -over-active imagination might be?", I asked with all the control I could muster.

"I know he just turned 60 'cause he has a couple of birthday cards on his desk congratulating him on turning 60," she said in her wee voice.

"You know he's full of beans, don't you?" We both laughed.

"Will you do me two favors, Marlene?" She was crying again. "Will you go to another oncologist? I know you said you'll have to drive further, but I think you'll understand that it's worth it. Also, will you not "play" that "tape" again in your mind of what this guy said to you? Throw it out, replace it with something else. Can you do that?"

"My children see me crying and they are so scared, I don't know what to tell them."

"Ask them to help you out. Ask them if it would be okay if every time you get this one thought in your mind, that you come up and give them a hug. Will you try these two things?"

Marlene said she would call me back in a couple of weeks and let me know how she was doing. Two days later I received a message asking me to call her back. That evening I reached her. In her meek voice, she shared with me what took place in the last 48 hours since we talked.

She found an oncologist who was 75 miles away. He took county payments, and he was even willing to see her in the evening after work. She went immediately to see him and his prognosis was not so grim. He suggested that she do only two cycles of chemotherapy, and then continue to be monitored every three months. His receptionist helped her apply for medical help from the county for chemotherapy.

This new oncologist also suggested she do acupuncture and herbal treatments at a clinic nearby.

Marlene sounded hopeful, and said she and her children were using the "hugging method" I had recommended to help relieve their stress. I was left with a promising image of a young woman, trusting herself and moving forward, instead of waiting for a "train" to come and run her down.

I called back over six months later. It was a Friday evening when her son answered the telephone and asked politely who was calling?

Marlene came to the telephone very excited. I was happy to hear her now strong voice and asked her to relay how things were going since our last conversation.

"I did the chemotherapy with very little problem. I also continue to do the acupuncture and herbs. In a month, the kids and I will be moving to a larger city and I will be attending college! I just received my high school diploma and I am very excited about the future!" Marlene was bubbling over. She lowered her voice and calmly said, "I can never thank you for what you said to me many months ago. It set the stage for everything that's happened to me, even with the cancer."

"I wish I could take credit for all of it,... maybe I'll take credit for controlling my temper when you told me about your first oncologist!" We both laughed and it was great "hearing" her "smile".

Marlene continued, "I remember lying in bed the evening when we talked. You told me to "replace the tape in my mind" of the oncologist telling me there was no hope. I thought about how much education he must have and how could he be wrong? I have very little education, but I remembered when I was in school, and the story of how people thought the world was flat many years ago. They even wrote it down in books and put it on maps, and anyone who thought differently was made fun of. I thought to myself, 'Marlene, you've made it this far on little judgment and little effort. What would happen if you made a big effort and trusted yourself, like... BIG TIME?' So that's what I did! The education will enable me to provide better for me and my kids."

I could not have been more proud of Marlene. A year later she revealed she was still attending school, still doing acupuncture, and continuing with follow-ups with her second oncologist.

Never ask "How long do I have?" Refuse to listen to someone's opinion on the date of your so-called demise. This is not denying the reality of your disease. If you devise a plan of action, that is the right one for you, the contrary opinion of one or a thousand people will not necessarily prove you wrong. If you believe in your own judgment, have researched your options, and are satisfied with your progress, then whatever people might think should not sway you.

Weigh criticism and listen to advice, but at the same time, gather wisdom by looking at those who are criticizing you as being fallible. After careful research go your own way, the way that is right for you. At the end of this book I have listed alternative resources. Don't stop there. Read other books which list conventional treatments. Keep one thing in mind when you are considering these resources or treatments. How does this <u>feel</u> to you?

Can you picture yourself successfully going through this treatment? Would the quality of your life be worth anything if you could not overcome the disease and your time here was short?

My healing came in part from my refusal to be treated like everyone else who had ovarian cancer. More than one person has told me that I was "in denial". It wasn't important what anyone wanted to call it. "Sticks and stones can break my bones but names can never hurt me."

My oncologist told me of my impending demise if I did not do extensive chemotherapy, and I knew at that moment that he would not be my "guide". He continued to harass me at home. He called me every day, never to ask "how are you feeling?", but asked if I had "changed my mind and come to my senses?" David was home one day when my oncologist called. He suggested my doctor willfully terminate our "relationship" or that we would do it legally.

There were many reasons why I chose to go to the Livingston Medical Center. One of the most important reasons was it "felt" good to be treated as an individual. There was not only one way to tame this ovarian cancer beast.

At the Livingston Center, several vials of blood were drawn on the first morning. Soon after, the doctor and the nutritionist got together with the lab and worked on what they believed was lacking in each person's blood, or what would benefit each person's immune system.

Many conventional medicine friends said "Hogwash" to Livingston's approach. They are not in my position nor do they understand every one's uniqueness.

A good example would be two individuals taking the exact same "cold medicine". A woman weighs 110 pounds and a man weighs 175 pounds. The woman experiences excessive drowsiness and needs to lie down for a few hours, while the man functions as usual.

This is a true example. I was that woman. I worked at an airport many years ago in Lake Tahoe. I was the unicom operator. The airport was a "non-controlled" airport which meant there was no FAA control tower, and I acted as an "advisory" for landings and takeoffs.

One late autumn day, I was advising traffic flying into the airport for the weekend. It was a very busy afternoon and I had a bad head cold. I complained about it to a friend of mine who was the 175 pound man, and he suggested I take two of his "cold" tablets.

I did as he prescribed and within 15 minutes I felt the effects of the medicine. I experienced extreme drowsiness and just wanted to find a warm place to lie down - not exactly the proper state of mind expected while guiding airplanes in or out of an airport. I was soon relieved of my duties by the "lineman", went home and did not return to normal until the next day.

This is a simplistic comparison to cancer treatments, but it is fitting. Another example was when I was at the Livingston Center. They do an intravenous Vitamin C treatment and attempt to get a person up to 45 grams per day. All along they remind you of the symptoms for when you have reached your body's maximum level. I leveled out at 20 grams. The other women with ovarian cancer took the maximum 45 grams per day.

Most of the people I have interviewed have complained about not being treated *individually* in conventional medicine. That is one of the reasons why they call me. I have never talked to anyone who likes their treatment or who is satisfied with their doctor. Those people are out there, but they never call me.

When I speak publicly, I have talked with people who don't care if they are treated individually. They are not interested in dealing with cancer uniquely or researching other options. We part company, respecting our individual right to treat our own disease.

You probably are not reading this book if you are perfectly

happy with what your doctor told you, or with your treatment. More than likely, you have designed your life to follow a more unique path. Continue on that path or create a new one. Healing is personal.

Do not commit to any procedure or treatment for at least 24 hours. Preferably longer. Give yourself time alone to think or meditate. Go away somewhere for a day or overnight. THERE ARE MANY ALTERNATIVES, even if that alternative is to do nothing for the time being.

CHAPTER SEVEN

Cancer generally gives us time. Time to work out the details in our life, time to tell people of our true thoughts, time to change. Even if we only have a few weeks, we have some time. Dropping dead from a heart attack is sudden and final and a shock for those loved ones left behind. Some people have told me they would prefer that sudden finality over having to deal with cancer and the many decisions that come with the disease. Of the people I have talked with most felt very lucky for at least having some time to "get real". Time to take care of unfinished business.

It becomes the perfect opportunity to part with people, things and environments that have been a cause for ill feelings. It is amazing how easily we can rid ourselves of these irritations when we have a different perspective of the fragility of our time on this Earth. Many found this to be their "favorite" experience in having cancer.

I remember talking with other people who had not experienced cancer or any life-threatening disease. Those dinner conversations when someone would say to me, "Micki, if I had cancer I would sell everything I had, pack my stuff and travel around the world!"

I remember hearing seminar speakers say "Take five minutes and write down everything you would do if you knew you only had six months to live." I would sarcastically write, "#1. If I knew I only had six months to live, then I must be God, so it wouldn't matter. #2. You're forgetting one thing. Most of the time you're very sick and really don't have the energy to cross the street." I was disappointed when I never got a reply on my scornful remarks. . .

Many people have a Hollywood version of how things will progress if they get a life-threatening disease. The movie opens with them racing around in their busy life. Then the bomb falls when they are told about the disease, sitting across from a Marcus Welby-type doctor. They ask the big question, "How long do I have?" The doctor grimaces and says, "If you're lucky, one year, but maybe three to four months. (You're the one who won't be lucky.) They run frantically from the doctor's office and get in their car and recklessly drive to the ocean. There they sit, sobbing uncontrollably until a seagull flies by and they have that moment of inspiration that we all believed would come to us. They return to their car, turn up the radio, wave to idle bystanders and arrive home, ready to share the news with loved ones. Only this time, they *know* what they must do. They sell all of their possessions or give them away and their neighbors think they are crazy. Soon they are off on a jetliner, visiting the Seven Wonders of the World. They return in the prescribed period of time to meet their demise. The last scene shows them lying in a hospital bed, dying alone. They decided to be like a wild animal and when the time came they went off on their own.

CHAPTER 7

There are many decisions to consider when deciding our cancer treatment path. Once we have heard our diagnosis, some people have very little time before they are pressured by their doctor to make a decision. Most of the time, if you are already in the hospital and you are set up with an oncologist, he has been making "plans" for your treatment before he even discusses it with you or your family members.

Many people are skeptical about alternative medicine. The same should happen with conventional medicine. Become an all-medicine skeptic. Even if you believe you will follow your doctor's advice to the end of the world, give yourself the time that this disease has allotted you.

David and I were amazed how quickly my oncologist had filled up my schedule with his recommended treatment. He never discussed it with us. He told us the way it would be.

One day when my oncologist came to see me in the hospital, he told me his plans for my treatment for the next two years. I said, "Hold on here. I feel like I'm buying a car. What's the hurry and the pressure?"

"You've got to commit to this chemotherapy treatment. You don't have time to fool around." He looked very serious. "This decision must be made today."

I do not remember saying, "Yes, I'll do chemotherapy". My silence <u>was</u> my decision. My oncologist assumed I would be doing the treatment. I assumed he assumed I had not made up my mind. Silence is not golden when it comes to saving your life. **SPEAK OUT !** Say, "I need time to think about this. When I feel I have figured it out, **I** will get back to **YOU !**"

The hundreds of people I interviewed have shared the pressure they felt from their doctors soon after their diagnoses. Their world was turned upside down and making such a vital decision seemed impossible for many of them.

Of the 500 people I interviewed, 175 made the decision to take some time and disappear for awhile. One man named Lance was sitting at his oncologist's desk with his wife at his side. They were discussing the chemotherapy treatments he would be taking for a year, followed by the radiation.

Lance said he just couldn't take it anymore and excused himself to use the bathroom. His wife remained in his oncologist's office. Lance did not go to the bathroom, but instead left the building, got in his car and drove across the street. He called his oncologist's office and had the nurse give his wife the message that he was waiting for her across the street.

Lance said he knew he should have faced his doctor and told him "NO", but he felt he was being pressured and his back was against the wall. His wife wanted him to do the chemotherapy and was taking sides with his oncologist.

Lance had colon cancer. After his episode at the oncologist's office, Lance went away for a week by himself to think things through. When he returned, his wife had told his doctor to go ahead and make plans to do the chemotherapy. By then Lance had already made his own plans. He had made an appointment to go to Livingston Medical Center. He came home to pack his bags and then left.

Lance had two years of touch and go with his cancer. He is now living in Mexico, retired and divorced.

A wonderful lady named Catherine told me a story similar to Lance's. After a five day hospital stay following her surgery to remove one breast, Catherine said she didn't like the sound of her doctor's advice - "Extensive radiation with a chemotherapy backup." She could not imagine participating in this program.

Dressed in hospital garb, Catherine grabbed her coat and told the nurse she was going out on the sun deck. She did not take her purse but stuffed her pockets with cash, credit cards and her driver's license. Outside of the hospital, Catherine hailed a cab and ended up at the Amtrak train station. The train ride to Los Angeles gave Catherine plenty of time to relax and think. When she arrived in Los Angeles still in her hospital "jammies", she sat in the train station for a couple of hours just watching the people. She tried to imagine what each person would do if they were in her situation. Several hours later, Catherine decided she should rent a car and drive the 550 miles back home. It took three days to drive back to her old life and along the way she called her boyfriend and explained her feelings. He was very upset and so was the hospital.

When Catherine arrived home she made many changes. She was a computer analyst in the Silicon Valley of California and she walked away from that life. She moved to the desert and pursued a life long dream of painting. Her boyfriend did not share her dream and they parted company.

Catherine pursued her own course of alternative healing. When we talked again over a year later, she was living and working in the Silicon Valley again. She said she was not as good of a painter as she thought, and she was lonely in the desert. She felt she had healed herself and has not shown any further signs of her previous disease.

Catherine had her hospital nightgown framed in a dramatic, carved-wooden frame that greets visitors when they walk into her enormous living room. Catherine titled it, "FUGITIVE IN FASHION", and entertains guests with her fascinating story.

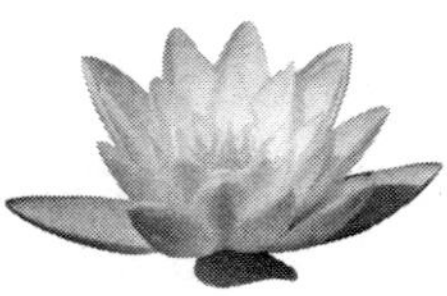

Giving yourself time to consider which treatment to choose is a healthy "cooling off" period. It allows you the chance to grieve and to gather support, if only from yourself. You cannot avoid your grief or anxiety, but you can support them if your mind is under control and if your thoughts are helpful. Map out your plan of action, and do your best to follow it. For sure your course will change as you learn more about yourself, your disease, and the research you have done.

Many people told me they were overwhelmed with the research they had done. When they discovered their options, they found it impossible to make a decision, or to settle on one treatment.

If you find yourself in this position, try taking a day, or several days and "disappear", even if you can't physically go somewhere.

Debbie called me in frustration. She had been researching alternative treatments for over a month. Her kitchen table was stacked with piles of notes, books and articles. Not knowing which way to turn, she asked me for some ideas.

My suggestion was probably not what she thought she would hear. "Leave it all alone for at least two days, preferably four or five days. Don't think about it, talk about it or sleep on it. Let it go. Your mind will let you know what is right for you. Give it time and space."

According to her oncologist, Debbie was "supposed" to be dead already. I was surprised by her reaction to my comments.

"You're right. What's another four or five days? I've already beat the deadline. My faith in God is strong and I guess with all of this clutter I'm just not able to hear His voice."

Debbie told me two months later that the "voice" she heard showed her the way. She didn't have much money, was a single mother of two children and very sick with Lung cancer. She went on to use Hydrazine Sulfate for her inoperable tumors and her pain. Debbie is still dealing with her cancer, but reminds me she is still hearing "the voice" and feels she is guided by God down the right path for her and her children.

How do you know what you are "feeling" is the right path of treatment? At this moment, you may be trying to answer that question. Or you may not have reached that point. Wherever you are in your research, you will most likely come to a place where you feel overwhelmed and frustrated. Like Debbie, you may have reached overload. The "cooling off" period helped Debbie get in touch with her "feelings", or "His Voice", as she put it.

The "feeling" might resemble one of weariness, a stress overload. If you give yourself time to separate from this monumental task, the "voice" of intuition (or God or the Universe) may have a chance to compete. When it looks like you just cannot take anymore, from somewhere an energy rises up. Every cell in your body feels replenished. Your mind becomes absolutely clear. At this moment you KNOW which way is best for you. Stay with that "feeling". Don't try to second-guess or analyze it. If you do, you have lost touch once again with that primitive knowing.

It is difficult for some people to understand that they must "feel" their way through this experience, not "think". Trying to "analyze" cancer will only get you bogged down in "data" and computer readouts. Would you be pleased to read about statistical data, or would you feel better to "talk" to or even "see" walking data?

My preference is the "walking" kind. Although each one of us is different, I appreciated seeing or talking with someone about their experience with a particular treatment. I wanted to "see" the whites of their eyes or hear their voices. Even in those early days when I first went to Livingston Medical Center, some of the people I met, who had returned for checkups, had several recurrences, or were still dealing with their cancer. It did not matter. They were as strong and healthy-looking as anyone you would know. More importantly, their personal power was in the right place. They were all dynamos. They knew where they were going and what they needed to do.

Many doctors spend a lot of time talking about data up to the "Five Year" period. That five year marker is used extensively by conventional medicine. Five minutes after midnight on the fifth year, someone could drop dead, but the data would list them as a long time survivor. That thinking has never inspired me. Why would you limit yourself to someone's statistical expectations?

Sometimes when I talk with people about having had cancer and they know I have not yet reached that infamous "five year" period, they say to me, "Well, that doesn't mean much until you've gone for five years without a recurrence". I retaliate with, "What am I, chopped liver? Who says it doesn't mean much?".

I know people do not make such a comment just to be mean. I thought the same way, and more than likely, said the same thing to someone many years ago. No one can understand the destruction of this statement until it is said to you. Maybe you just "gotta be there".

Waiting for that five year period is very destructive. The disappointment of not making it to the fifth year creates anxiety, terror and a sense of letting your loved ones down. Many people have agonized over their let down and told me it was worse than originally finding out they had cancer. Do not put yourself through this emotional roller-coaster! Even if the rest of the world wants to believe it, you do not have to. You know the world is ROUND!

You can not change other peoples' beliefs, but you can change your own. Do not spend your time trying to change what someone else wants to cling to. Until they are walking in your moccasins, they are comforted by a mass conviction.

We can turn on the television or radio and see the "mass conviction" alive and well. It is called advertising. If we think we are immune because we are smarter, then I have a bridge to sell to you in San Francisco. Recently, I saw an ad on TV that was selling a medical treatment in a cortisone cream. One of the statements in the ad went like this, "Did you know that you can still get poison oak for up to one year if wearing the same unwashed clothes ?" (If you're wearing the same unwashed clothes after a year, you deserve poison oak !). Pay attention to the first part, "you can still get poison oak for up to one year". What happens if you wear those clothes 13 months instead of 12 months later ? Is there really a time limit with the resin from poison oak?

This statement was well-researched and cost the company lots of money, word for word. Soon after I became aware of this "message", I saw a friend of mine in the drug store buying this particular product for her daughter's poison oak. She said she "heard on tv" that it worked.

Before I end this chapter, I would like to take this "decision" one step further. If you are an adult with cancer, you have every legal right to commit or not commit to a procedure. In most States, a practitioner (whether in conventional or alternative medicine) must inform you that chemotherapy or radiation are the "legal"treatments for cancer. Every other alternative is just that and is used to "boost the immune system".

Of the people who called me, several told me of difficulties they had being released from the hospital or their doctor's care, because they did not agree to go along with chemotherapy or radiation. In a few incidences, tempers flared and they had to take drastic measures to get themselves or their loved one out of the grips of the hospital.

A prominent man from Dallas, Texas told me how he asked for his very ill wife to be released from the hospital, and with her consent he could take her to another facility. The hospital told him she was not fit to be moved and that they would not release her. This man is well-known in the Dallas area and called the police to get his own personal escort to retrieve his wife. She ended up dying two months later, but it was on her terms.

I have talked to lawyers who were familiar with this subject. They have said that anyone over the age of 18 has the right to refuse any treatment. That right does not extend to children. I have spoken to five people who had children with cancer who were under the legal age. Three of the five stories were devastating for the whole family, including the child.

In those three cases, the families had attempted to escape to other countries to get their child treated. Only one family successfully accomplished this and now lives in Costa Rica. Their son is in remission from leukemia. This family cannot return to the United States until the boy is of legal age. They were told by their lawyer, that if their son dies before age eighteen and they return to the United States, they will be up for murder charges! They left family, a house, and their belongings to escape before Child Protective Services stepped in and could return the boy to the hospital, and to the chemotherapy which the parents thought was killing him.

In two of the other cases, the parents attempted to flee with their child, but were caught, treated like criminals, and only allowed to see their child under the supervision of Child Protective Services. Both children died within six months of chemotherapy treatments.

I asked one of the parents whose child died while in chemotherapy treatment, what they would have done differently? The mother said she would never have brought him back to the doctor where the boy's first blood test was taken. She said they would have quietly "disappeared" and treated him alternatively.

The anguish each one of these parents felt was heartbreaking. The decision to do what they thought would be best for the child was overridden by the law.

When I asked the mother why she felt chemotherapy was killing her son, she told me they found in their research that childhood "leukemia" was shown in many cases to be "outgrown". In those cases, complicated treatments were not done. It was treated by boosting the immune system with healthy food and rest.

In continued research on childhood leukemia, they read about the effects of chemotherapy. The child may recuperate and the leukemia may go into remission. Ten years later it may rear its ugly head again in another form of cancer.

These have to be the most heart wrenching stories. It is tragic when cancer takes up residence in the body of an adult. When it is a child, no one can imagine anything more devastating. If you have children it is prudent to stop for one minute and consider the decision you might make. You will not have the "luxury" of choosing a treatment. That decision will already have been made for you - it is the law!

CONSIDER ALL OPTIONS. You are like a hub in a wheel. The spokes are the people and treatments that will be helping you. Your doctor is only one of those spokes.

CHAPTER EIGHT

Once you realize that your doctor, and his recommended treatments, are only the tip of the iceberg in dealing with cancer, you will feel like you have been released from solitary confinement. There is a "world" within the world of cancer. Albeit overwhelming, still it is there and functioning. My suggestion is to dip your toe in the spring of information available to you and continue to test the waters. If you don't feel comfortable just jumping in, then go in up to your knees and seek out something minor in the alternative field for a start.

The metaphor of the wheel - you are the hub and the people and treatments are the spokes - was told to me by a man named Ken. I loved the idea! It gave me a clear, concise image of how I needed to function and maintain my life.

Ken had AIDS. When we talked he had very little time left in his quest. His "Killer Cells" were down to four. The way he dealt with his "wheel" could give anybody an empowering course of action. Ken drew a large picture of a wheel with a hub with spokes to balance it. He wrote his name on the hub, then wrote individual people and treatments on each spoke. He said the number of spokes changed frequently as he added treatments or took them away. After using a paper wheel for a time, he had a friend design a sophisticated cut-out wheel that he kept on his kitchen wall. He even had broken spokes to indicate the treatments, doctors, or people who needed to be replaced. Until he could replace them with some other form of treatment or person, he left the broken spoke in the wheel. This gave him time to consider who would be the substitute without feeling overwhelmed. It also gave him a larger picture of his arrangement. I thought his idea ingenious!

Just before Ken died 8 months later, he called to "will" me his wheel idea.

The metaphor of the wheel extends further. Our ancestors depended on the wheel, literally and figuratively, even more than we do today. They depended on the wheel as a whole. If one spoke broke, they either replaced it, or went as far as they could before they could work on it. It was their lifeblood, their way of surviving.

Figuratively, their "wheel" represented the people and medicines that helped them survive. Their doctor or medicine man was only one of those spokes. They could not and did not depend solely on him. Maybe you are not interested in reinventing the Wild West. Maybe you believe that with all of the technology that we have today, all you have to do is have "someone else take care of it for you". If you take the time to do your "wheel" you might find this to be true. Is that "someone" doing a good job with your disease? Despite the condition of your disease, do you feel like you are being treated with dignity, kindness and individuality? Are you sure that your treatment will be covered entirely by your insurance company? And if not, will you have to file for bankruptcy?

Some names to put on your "spokes" are as follows : INSURANCE, DOCTORS (OR MEDICINE MEN OR WOMEN), TREATMENTS, CAREGIVERS, PETS, LIVING WILL, HEALERS, SPIRITUAL, HUMOR, SANCTUARIES, CELEBRATIONS, etc.

Here are some examples of how these "spokes" can affect your life.

INSURANCE: What a gigantic can of worms. How can I write about this monolith in a few paragraphs? What's the definition of insurance, I ask? Mr. Webster says, "Insurance, 1. an insuring or being insured against loss. 2. a contract whereby, in return for a fixed payment (premium), the insurer guarantees the insured that a certain sum will be paid for a specified loss: usually called insurance policy." Does this sound like your insurance?

It might if you were talking about fire, property, earthquake or even life insurance. How about your medical, or "health" insurance? Your health is your loss. The part that states " a <u>certain</u> sum will be paid for a <u>specified</u> loss" is critical. It is open to interpretation, but accurate, and very much what the insurer is counting on. I see how open to interpretation this definition is and how it affects each one of us. The battle between the insured and the insurer is in full force. Still most people will not feel the force of that battle until they get involved in a life-threatening disease or catastrophic situation.

Every person who calls me, at one time or another, deals with the issue of insurance - whether they have it or not. The stories I have heard are tragic and relentless. On the subject of insurance, I tell people who call me "if you have it, PRETEND LIKE YOU DON'T !" When I say that, many reply smugly, "I'm well covered."

What appears to be called "good" insurance is based on coverage of anything and the numbers to back that anything. This is a big mistake. Each of the 501 people I interviewed (I've included myself !) discovered that healing is not based on a numbers game, a probability game, or any game. "Good" insurance gives you NO BETTER CHANCE OF SURVIVAL from cancer than no insurance! Being "well covered" does nothing for increasing your chances of survival. I know this first hand. I DID NOT AND DO NOT HAVE HEALTH INSURANCE ! I am not endorsing that you drop your insurance, for me it was a part of my fate.

A surgical operation and several nights in a hospital can certainly damage the pocketbook. It would have destroyed me if I did not have loyal and devoted family and friends. Because of them, I did have the choice for continuing chemotherapy. I chose not to. At times I have wondered, was I lucky not to have insurance?

It is not the American way to live without health insurance. Those of us that do not have it are considered to be the unfortunate ones. I would agree, if we are talking about a car accident or falling out of a tree. Emergency room fees are astronomical.

I think it is a different picture with disease. No insurance and a diagnosis of cancer would be to most people, a fate worse than death. Not true!

Of course it is scary. Of course you start looking for some great aunt to take mercy on you and cover you financially. But when you are spending your own money, you spend it carefully. You research carefully. You make your decisions carefully. You are less likely to do chemotherapy or radiation and more likely to do alternative medicine.

Many doctors object to alternative medicine. They feel that many who work in this field take advantage of very ill people. Doctors believe that the patient's money is being squandered. The patient is duped and left with nothing. In my own case, the opposite was true.

When you don't have health insurance, you become a creative genius in the areas of your healing. You are less likely to waltz into an environment, conventional or alternative, and say "I don't care what it costs, give it to me". People with health insurance have a better chance of being dazzled by a mere promise. They pay their premiums and they expect the service. It is not important how much that "service" costs; they are not interested. To believe the higher the price, the better the service, is absurd. I am still around to prove it!

This is not a condemnation of insurance companies or agents. I am simply suggesting that you question your doctor, hospital, and insurance coverage. Question the cost of treatment and do your homework.

Diane called me from Seattle, Washington. She had ovarian cancer and was just finishing up her sixth month of chemotherapy. Her cancer had not been thwarted. She was seeking an alternative treatment and facing the cost. The average price was $10,000 to $15,000. She said paying that amount out of her pocket would be difficult and she wondered how "alternative medicine could be so incredibly expensive?"

Diane was "well covered" with medical insurance. She paid a very minimal deductible. I knew she had absolutely no idea how much her six months of chemotherapy cost the insurance company. I asked, "How much did your chemotherapy cost?".

"Nothing. I'm well covered," she said smugly.

"I know that, but let's look at this in a different light. Go back to your oncologist and ask for a readout of the cost of your treatments in the last six months. Ask him to include his office fees, hospital fees and drug fees." Diane took my suggestion and called me back two weeks later. She was flabbergasted. The total billed to her insurance company was $210,000.00 for six months of chemotherapy.

"Do you think it was worth it?" I asked.

"Not if I'm still shopping around!" she replied.

If she used alternative medicine, there are no guarantees that Diane would have done any better with her cancer. We both agreed on that. We did agree that she might have had a better quality of life. We will never know. Diane died six weeks later.

Because chemotherapy, surgery and radiation are the only legal and "respected" treatments for cancer (in the United States only), and are recognized by the Food and Drug Administration, insurance companies will pay that exorbitant amount. That is changing.

Randi called me for the third time before we discussed her insurance dilemma. She had always paid her policy promptly but was now faced with a bill for a second round (4 months) of radiation. The bill was for $42,000! Her insurance company refused to pay this bill because two years earlier she had done chemotherapy and radiation for over a year. Randi had breast cancer and it was advancing. Her doctor suggested a newer form of radiation and she went ahead with the procedure, not thinking to check with her insurance company beforehand. She assumed she would be covered, and so did the hospital. Randi discovered the insurance company did not approve of this new form of radiation, and said Randi would be responsible for the entire bill! When we last talked she was making monthly payments of $410.

I have talked to other people who have had as much chemotherapy as their insurance would allow. Many companies are now putting a two year limit on paying for these treatments. The usual scenario is the doctor will suggest the person stay on the chemotherapy until the insurance company says "that's enough; we won't cover this anymore." Then the doctor tells the patient they have come to the end of the line and there is nothing more they can do.

A very angry man named Preston told me his tale of woe. I was not sure if he was angry at the doctors, his insurance company, or both. He called it his "use you, then lose you" theory.

"They use your money, make it look like they're concerned about you, then one day, you get the axe and they're on to someone else. Sounds like prostitution to me!" Preston was indignant. Preston did chemotherapy until his insurance company called "foul". At the same time his doctor told Preston that there was nothing more that he could do for him. By now Preston's body was sick and ravaged by chemotherapy, and he was also having a difficult time finding an alternative center that would take him. For many this becomes another frightful experience. People have discovered that if they do too much chemotherapy or radiation, their alternative choices dwindle to a few. Some have reached a point where their bodies are so ravaged, there is very little hope being offered. Never let that experience get you down! There will always be "something" that will provide for you a glimmer of hope or a chance to make your final days more satisfying.

Some people have told me, "What does it matter how much it cost my insurance company? I have paid my premiums; they need to live up to their end of the bargain." As a person who does not have insurance, I can see how this attitude leads to where we are today. Insurance companies will constantly keep raising premiums if people are never concerned about the cost or effectiveness of their treatments. Most importantly, is there a better treatment for you, and because your insurance company will not cover it, you do not try it? This is your life, and unless you are a cat, it is probably the only life you are going to have, in this dimension anyway! Why would you ignore other possibilities because your policy does not cover them?

Some people have displayed bizarre behavior in the name of "benefits". I have talked to people who have remained in jobs they hated because the "benefits" were good. "Is your life good?" I would ask. "It doesn't matter," they would tell me. They wanted security for their families in case "something happened". Well, something did happen and now they had reached the limit of their insurance policy, and still had to find money to cover a treatment their insurance policy would not cover.

I heard from Anne one day after a whole week of hearing insurance stories. Anne said she had an 80% coverage on her policy. She had done 5 months of chemotherapy before the bills caught up with her. She never bothered to ask how much her treatment was. "How expensive could chemotherapy drugs be?" she naively thought to herself. Anne found out. Her 5 months of chemotherapy totaled $180,000.00. With Anne's insurance coverage, she was left to pay 20% or $36,000.00! She had 3 more months of chemotherapy. Anne had to drop out of the treatments. She now was in debt, still had cancer and was seeking other options which were hopefully, less expensive and more effective.

The experiences of Diane, Randi, Preston and Anne are not very healing when you have cancer. Each one was very sick. Each had to deal with their insurance company, the possibility that their doctor would give up on them, and the pain and agony of their treatments. Each had no idea if she would survive!

No matter what treatment we choose, there are no absolutes to getting better or returning to life as we once knew it. We <u>can</u> help ourselves by researching and studying <u>all</u> options beyond what our insurance company will cover. In the long run, we may be paying more out-of-pocket, or we may be cut off from any more insurance-covered treatments, only to find ourselves gravely ill and searching for another alternative.

This may be a fantasy, but hopefully one day we will be given the option of "insurance menu policies". If we were not using conventional medicine, like myself, we could still have the option for accident or emergency care coverage.

The United States is one of the best countries in the world for trauma care. We learned a lot about triage and traumatic injuries from the Vietnam War. Soon after, trauma centers as we know them today, sprung up in major cities across this country.

When it comes to disease our score has been poor. Not much has changed, except for the dramatic <u>increase</u> of cancer in the last twenty years. If you have insurance, USE IT LIKE YOU DO NOT HAVE IT!

DOCTORS (OR MEDICINE MEN OR WOMEN):

Use a doctor for disease LIKE YOU DON'T HAVE ONE! I know that sounds odd, but a doctor should be used only for consultation for a disease. Use his knowledge for what he knows, then consult with someone else or somewhere else for further knowledge. This makes many people uncomfortable because they want to have a "relationship" with their doctor. That "relationship" is fine if you and your doctor belong to the Rotary Club, but your disease will require many consultations with many different people.

Use your wheel. Doctors are just one of the many spokes. Your health is what is of primary importance; you are the hub. The spokes are to work in unison, together, FOR YOU! If one of those spokes is demanding to replace you as the hub, REPLACE THEM! As my grandmother used to tell me, "There are plenty of "spokes" in the sea!"

In this country we are very narrow-minded when it comes to healing. Because a doctor is schooled for 8 to 12 years we believe they will walk out with the ability to cure us for anything from a cold to cancer. We adorn them with a title which gives them instant respect and power. Mention "doctor" and visions of financial success buzz through our head.

There are many doctors worth their weight in gold. Truly helpful and compassionate people. But you must consider how you are treated by your doctor. If they have become the biggest part of your life, then my belief is you will need to either replace them or balance out your "wheel".

When people are infatuated with their doctors, they relinquish their own power. People tell me about drugs they are using, recite technical jargon, and the hopelessness of their disease, as told by their doctor. I usually cut in somewhere and ask a simple question. "When does the healing start?"

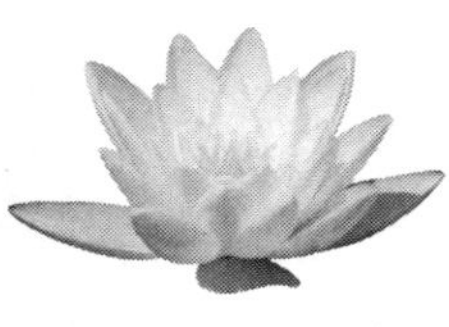

Margo sounded like she worked for a pharmaceutical company

when she chattered on about her disease. She had ovarian cancer. I let her continue. She listed six different drugs she was taking along with the chemotherapy and four over-the-counter drugs to counteract the effects of the other drugs. I asked her to tell me how she spent her day. Between two naps a day, she was on the phone with her doctor, hospital, insurance company, pharmacists and several friends she felt she could "bleed on"(her words, not mine).

I asked her the inevitable question, "When does the healing start?" "Well, my doctor says <u>if</u> I am cured, it probably won't be for quite awhile." She said that as nonchalantly as you read it.

I have met and talked with many people like Margo who "parrot" their doctor's every word. They spend their days and nights living their disease. This is not the doctor's fault; he is focused on hundreds of other patients that he sees. Margo made herself dependent on her doctor and the assembly of people <u>she</u> supported. I heard nothing from Margo about healing.

The energy Margo put into analyzing her situation could have been spent with the "spokes" that would be supporting <u>her.</u> If she appreciated her doctor for his knowledge, I would find that acceptable. Instead, she clung to his every word. She needed to balance his negative attitude with those who might suggest that Margo get on with her life.

"Healing" is a word not commonly used by doctors. They like the word "cure". Cure indicates more long-term, scientific terminology. Test your doctor. Count how many times he uses the word "heal" versus "cure". If "healing" is used to describe his ultimate goal for you, you might consider coming back. Why does that matter ? Borrowing from Mr. Webster, a "cure" is a remedy, a system or method of <u>medical</u> treatment. A "healing" is to make sound, well or healthy again; to restore to health; **to free from grief and troubles.** A cure is generally pursued through a program or a method. A healing is an intangible or an abstract process. Most doctors could not imagine "healing someone of cancer". They prefer to "cure someone of cancer". My oncologist told me I "would never be cured of cancer". Not a very optimistic note, but I did not care. It was not important to me to be "cured". I wanted to be "healed".

I prefer the "healing" method. It happens NOW. It means I live my life, whatever time I have, NOW. "Curing" indicates waiting, like "curing" meat. Both "healing" and "curing" take time, but with "healing" you do what needs to get done concerning your health, and you still have time each day for a life! You move from the threat and horrific experience of learning you have cancer, to healing and living.

Like Margo, you could wait around for your doctor to let you know when you are cured. That is like waiting to win the lottery! You put your life on hold and fantasize what might be.

If Margo had declared herself "to be healing" her mind and her body would already be starting the process. Just because you intend something does not always make it so, but if you are "restoring your health and are free from grief and troubles", then you are "healed" !

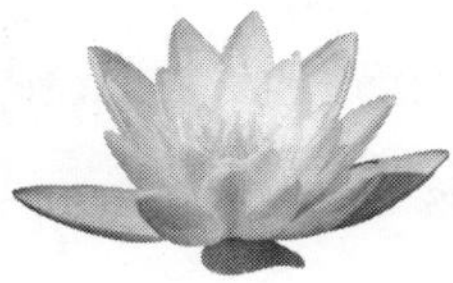

TREATMENTS: In my thinking, your treatment for cancer should not consume your life. If you are very ill, it still should not be your main focus.

When I did one cycle of chemotherapy, I felt consumed by it. It was not only the physical detriment of what health I had left, but it was focusing on the cancer, not the healing. Somehow, my body allowed the cancer to proliferate. Somehow I would find a way to reverse that process. Not with chemotherapy.

Everyone has the right to choose their form of treatment without ridicule from anyone, including doctors. On your wheel spokes, I hope you will list many treatments. When I have asked about what "treatment" they are using, most people brought up their doctors and the standardized cancer treatments.

You have the right to choose or refuse any treatment. Some treatments are not legal in the United States, if you find this to be the treatment that you prefer then fly off to wherever that treatment is being used. Prepare to change your treatments as you change your life. Use the Resource Guide at the end of this book to explore alternative clinics, doctors and tests. Calling is cheap when compared to your life.

If you choose the standardized, conventional treatments for cancer - surgery, chemotherapy and radiation - research and read all that you can on those subjects. Just before I did chemotherapy, I was given several pages to read about what can happen while the drugs are being administered, and possible effects in the future. Chills went up my spine. Chemotherapy is a known carcinogen, sometimes creating its own cancer. It can also cause a stroke, heart attack, seizures, and internal bleeding, just to name a few of the side effects.

I remember the oldest woman out of the 500 people I interviewed. Her name was Heloish which she said was Yiddish for "brave". Heloish was more then brave, she was hell-on-wheels. After her second bout with ovarian cancer, Heloish formed her own "club". She called it the Bubu Club (which is Yiddish for mistake). Heloish recruited club members by visiting hospitals and oncologists' offices to find other cancer patients.

She passed out a booklet she typed up and printed herself. The booklet was titled, *THE GREAT BUBU*. In the booklet, Heloish condemned the present standardized treatments of cancer. She wrote out facts and statistics, and just plainly wrote what a big "bubu" or mistake someone was making in taking these treatments. Her booklet was filled with lengthy reports on the misuse of chemotherapy and radiation. Heloish knew she was an annoyance, but said everyone treated her kindly, even though she was stealing their patients. Heloish was 81 years young when we met at a small gathering where I was speaking. I would never have believed she was her age. She looked ten years younger. I asked her what she said when she walked up to a possible recruit, and did she expect a negative reaction?

"Oh never ! Besides, I'm hard of hearing, so most of the time I probably don't really hear what they say to me. I just smile a lot and they smile back. I approach someone, introduce myself, and hand them my booklet. I'm not asking them for anything. I don't want money. I don't want them to leave with me. I just ask them to read the booklet and decide on their own. My "club" does not have a phone number, just a post office box. Once a week I pick up my mail and it's overflowing with letters. People just go through the motions until someone shows them another way - *gently*." I smiled as she put her hands together as in prayer and bowed her head. Then she looked up at me and said, "Once people read my booklet, they figure out that this cancer thing isn't all it's cracked up to be anyway! They get brave and get some "chutzpah" (Yiddish for gall) and get on with what life they have left!"

Heloish did change a lot of lives. After her death at age 83, her daughter called to talk with me. Heloish had lived with her daughter, Christine. Christine told me when cleaning out Heloish's belongings, she gathered all of the letters that people had written to her mother and the Bubu Club. There were over 5,000 letters! Each one of those people wrote to tell Heloish that they were "saved" by her booklet, and they went on to do optional treatments. I could hear the pride for her mother when she told me at Heloish's funeral about the hundreds of people that came and left notes eulogizing this "heloish" woman.

Five years after my experience with cancer, I still continue with the Livingston program. I eat as healthy as I can, but I have never made food the center of my life. I do well with juicing, especially with vegetables. I juice vegetables and eat fruit. That is not the best way to consume my daily needs, but it works for me. The rule I give myself is to eat 60 to 80% of my daily intake as "live food". I told that to a caller one day who said, "Well, I already do that. I'm a big meat eater !" When I mentioned to her that the meat she is eating is actually dead, and that live food had helpful enzymes in it, she snapped at me and said, "If you're a vegetarian, then how do you know whether meat does or does not have enzymes in it?"

"You're right, I don't know," I said and ended the conversation quickly. Sometimes our best medicine is to know when to strike like the rattlesnake, or when to retreat!

I also take a short nap each day, hike twice a day with my dogs and do tai chi or other exercises. After my nap, I chant for 20 minutes. Besides the handful of vitamins and minerals I take daily, I use my Rife instrument 3 to 4 times a week. What is a Rife instrument? It's an electromagnetic device using bio-active frequencies. I use it for everything from poison oak, allergies, back pain to boosting my immune system. It was invented by the scientist, Royal Raymond Rife, who spent two decades studying the unique electromagnetic "signature" of viruses, bacteria and fungi and experimented with special frequencies to destroy them. For further information call the company listed in the Resource Guide under RIFE INSTRUMENT.

Besides the regimen above, my other "treatments" are my work, my solitude, my daily laughter and my healthy relationships. If your relationships are not healthy and you don't feel that you can remove yourself from them as yet, CREATE new relationships that are beneficial and invigorating. The unhealthy ones will soon go to the wayside.

Cancer treatments need to give you the balance of the physical, mental and spiritual. If you are only concerned with the physical aspect of cancer, then the balance is not happening. That is true for the mental and the spiritual, also.

Arlene told me she healed herself by prayer alone. She described her experience and her everyday life to me. The prayer started as her main focus. It was her treatment. What she did not see was how the prayer opened up her mind. She was more accepting of others in her life. She also had become more physically active, going on hikes three times a week with other people in her prayer group. They all shared their healthy eating habits. Prayer led her to Christian concerts where she met a gentleman who she is now dating. Despite the seriousness of her breast cancer, Arlene created a new life. Her prayer-power was her primary treatment, which eventually led to many other treatments.

Many people believe that the only way we will ever find a "cure" for cancer is by putting up more money for research. I halfway agree with that, but the other half of me believes that most of the research being done today is wrapped up in the use of pharmaceutical drugs. Good health comes from the organic farm, not from your local pharmacy !

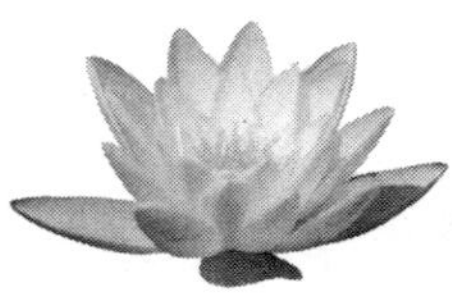

CAREGIVERS: "As the sun illuminates the moon and the stars, so let us illumine one another." -Anonymous

Caregivers come in many shapes and sizes and from the oddest places in our lives. A woman named Margaret called me one rainy day, asking for information on alternative treatment centers - in sunny climates. She was from Chicago and was taking care of a young woman in her mid-thirties. The young woman's name was Candy. Margaret told me that she just celebrated her 70th birthday. She wanted to take Candy to some sort of a treatment center where she would be able to feel the sun and hopefully watch the ocean. Candy had ovarian cancer, a very advanced stage.

After discussing the Livingston Center in San Diego and a few centers in Mexico, I asked Margaret if she and Candy were related.

"Not really. I knew Candy's father very well." Margaret paused for a few seconds, "Actually, to be honest with you, I had a 20 year affair with Candy's father." I was at a loss for words until Margaret broke the moment. "Candy's parents divorced about five years ago and I don't know if it was because of my affair with her father, Don. Last year, both Don and his ex-wife died within three months of each other. I heard that Candy, who never married, was diagnosed with cancer soon after her parents died. I thought, "What else could happen to this poor girl?" So I called Candy and went to see her. We have become fast friends ever since. She is not aware of my indiscretion with her father. She just thinks I'm a close family friend."

Margaret went on to tell me that at first, her visits stemmed from her guilt, but soon she felt total love and compassion for Candy. They were living together when we talked. Candy's health was deteriorating quickly. She had done almost a year of chemotherapy until her white blood count started to elevate.

Margaret was using her own money to care for Candy, and to

cover many of her medical expenses, outside of what was being covered by Candy's insurance.

Margaret and Candy settled on Dr. Donsbach's facility in Rosarita Beach, Mexico. Candy enjoyed her brief stay in the sun before she died in Margaret's arms. Candy had no other relatives - except her loyal friend, Margaret.

Most of the caregivers I talk with have not chosen the task, as in Margaret's case. It just happened. Most of them were spouses, close relatives, or live-ins.

I find it best if you can have several caregivers in your life. Each one good at one task, and of course, each one sharing ideas, and occasionally challenging those ideas.

I call them "foxhole buddies". Although I am adverse to using war terminology with cancer healing, a "foxhole buddy" is a fitting term and they are easy to identify. Who would you want in your foxhole when the proverbial "stuff" hits the fan? If you have more buddies than you can fit in a Volkswagen, then rethink your foxhole. More is not better. Quality is what you want and the role each one plays in your life.

My husband David was given the task of caregiving for me. He juggled his life, and mine, and still offered his support and love. He was the perfect caregiver although I was not the perfect patient!

I also had several members of my family and close friends. There are also the "temporary caregivers". They stroll in and out of your life and offer support, but generally, it is on their terms and whenever they can fit you into their schedule.

When asked about their caregivers, each person told me that they did not find it hard to remove someone from their lives if they could not get along. Even if that person was married to them, related or a close friend.

Sometimes people were faced with the opposite problem. Who they thought would be their caregivers, ended up leaving them, sometimes at the moment they were told the news of their cancer. I have heard this most commonly from women who had breast cancer. Out of the 34 women I have talked with who had breast cancer, 22 were married or living with a partner, and an alarming 13 of those 22 women watched their partners walk out the door!

In the last year, I have seen an interesting trend developing with caregivers. Many siblings have served as caregiver. For example, several women I have talked with have their single brothers acting as their guardians. It is always delightful to talk with these sensitive, but determined men. They have tremendous compassion, strong wills and the ability to seize the situation when the need arises. The same applies to sister siblings, cousins and even children. Being in my late forties, I am always surprised to talk with the 20 year old "children" of people my age.

If you have several trusting caregivers, their lives will not be as hectic. We must understand, through our pain and fear, that they must carry on with parts of their existence. I have talked with and seen caregivers who have reached their breaking point. They are stressed and physically ill themselves. The Livingston Medical Center suggests that the caregiver come to the center with the patient. They will usually do a blood test on the caregiver to see their state of health, and they encourage them to participate in parts of the program.

I often thought how much easier it was for me, the person with the disease, than for David. I knew what I was thinking, when I was fearful or anxious. David had to always wonder or try to imagine what I must have been going through. Sometimes, he probably thought I was afraid and worried, when I was just dealing with gas pains, or thinking about what I might eat that evening that would not give me gas! The job of caregiver is difficult.

I remember a short poem a woman slipped to me at one of my talks. She scratched it on a torn piece of paper without signing her name.

It goes: "I gathered friends like fields of daffodils, assuming they would always be there. When the time came and I was ill, the one's who did care, were from that same field of daffodils, but they were just a pair."

PETS: One of my favorite spokes on the wheel is pets. They should be included as caregivers, but they deserve a heading all of their own. I have had many pets in my life. They did not keep me from getting cancer, but they were instrumental in my healing from it.

The day I came home from the hospital, after my cancer surgery and diagnosis, I was surrounded by my pets. Their unconditional love, their devotion, and their way of living in the present, were all I needed as a welcoming committee.

I believe animals have the ability to cross over to other dimensions. They feel and see things that we are incapable of doing with our logical minds. I have had dogs that have warned me of danger ahead of time. I was saved by my puppy, Otis, who was only five months old. He licked my face until I woke up in a rainstorm, after being knocked out by a tree I had cut down.

I believe my dog Tonto knew I had cancer during the days of going from doctor to doctor. He sacrificed his life two months before my surgery, to make me aware of the danger I was in. (That is another book!) It has been found that some dogs can sniff out cancer. Others can tell if someone is going to have a seizure and warn the person before it happens.

Over half of the people I talked with had a pet that they relied on for companionship and part of their healing. Many people said having a pet made them do things each day, like feeding them or taking them for a walk. My dogs have to be walked every day, twice a day, even when I am not in the mood. They always are and so are my cats.

In the days before I knew I had cancer, but was supporting a "fibroid" tumor, I experienced excruciating pain. I believe I would easily have given up and just curled up and died, if it was not for my pets. My dogs were willing to stay with me even if I did not walk them, but their enthusiasm was contagious and uplifting when they saw me put on my shoes. Running back and forth through the house, barking with such glee, how could your spirits not be lifted from such a simple act?

My pets have helped me forget my misery. They have known just the right moment to plant a slobbering kiss on my face or rub against my leg.When I have felt stressed and under pressure, I have learned to keep cadence with their breathing while they are napping. The times I have fallen short on my daily requirement of laughter, I will listen to their snorting and snoring or chase one or more of them around the yard.

If you do not have a pet or do not feel like you can make a commitment to one, you can always volunteer to help out at your local animal shelter. One or two days a week, you can walk dogs or groom cats. These animals are in need of human contact, being confined in a small cage day after day.

I hope you will not get a pet just to satisfy your emotional needs. If you really do not know if you want to commit to having one, or you can not provide for it while you are here, or after you die, rent a video on animals instead, or go to the zoo. Pets deserve your commitment, do not let them down.

LIVING WILL: We can extend our commitment to our pets after we die by making a will. Put together a plan to financially provide for them and specify someone or someplace where they will be cared for after our death.

If you do not have the money to leave for the care of your pets, then create a network of friends, family, or co-workers and work with them to help you arrange for the proper treatment for your pets after you die. If you cannot afford to retain a lawyer for your "estate planning", at least create a will that will express your wishes and how you have planned to care for the lives you have shared.

I knew a woman who was very active in our local animal shelter. She had over 30 dogs and cats on her ranch. She made these animals the center of her life. She died suddenly of an infection. We were all shocked. Her pets had to be taken to the animal shelter. Some had to be euthanized because they were too weak and ill to make a change. The animal shelter was strapped for funds and short of room after all of her pets were taken in. This devoted steward of animals left no will or plan for her pet's future. Her estate was left to a friend who lived on the property. He made no contribution to the provision of this woman's beloved friends. Never assume people around you will handle your affairs the way you think they might.

Beyond pets, a living will should be made to dispense with your "stuff". As many of us have seen or heard, people's behavior changes when there is money or property to be inherited. Sometimes it can be an ugly scene.

Besides your property and possessions, you should go beyond a living will. The Commission on Aging with Dignity in Tallahassee, Florida is a non-profit, private, charitable organization. They have devised the FIVE WISHES Living Will. They describe their FIVE WISHES as follows: "We have found that current living wills, which look only at the medical needs of those seriously ill, no longer are sufficient. People who are seriously ill want to be treated with dignity, and they are concerned about family forgiveness, reconciliation, and relief from physical pain, if and when it comes. FIVE WISHES gives you the opportunity to make all of your wishes known, and to have your God-given dignity respected."

Presently, FIVE WISHES Living Will is only legal in the state of Florida, but the Commission on Aging With Dignity is working to make it legal in other states. You can write the Commission at the address listed under "Living Wills" in the Resource Guide. Ask for a copy of the FIVE WISHES and you might include a charitable donation since they receive no government money.

Many people assume that if they just write in their will that they do not want "to be hooked up to any tubes or machines," that they do not have to say more. In the conversations I have had with many caregivers, just writing that statement does not relieve them of the burden. How about pain medication? Is morphine for you, or would you prefer other alternatives like Hydrazine Sulfate? Depending on the quantity of morphine, some people are rarely lucid, and drift in and out of their semi-conscious state. I have talked with many people who have taken Hydrazine Sulfate and felt a sense of euphoria, and at least were able to share a conversation with their loved ones before they died. The protocol of Hydrazine Sulfate must be strictly adhered to, otherwise your pain can worsen. If you have the Internet available to you, keyword "Hydrazine Sulfate" and you will come up with hundreds of web sites.

The process of dying from a disease is, at times, a complicated one. Do your caregiver a big favor and spell out just what you do or do not want. They will be able to deal with your departure much better and not feel like they have failed you.

An example is a story of a woman named Lesley. Her live-in boyfriend of seven years was dying of cancer when Leslie called me. She was hanging onto threads of hope. We talked about the problem she was having with her boyfriend's grown children. Lesley broke down and cried. Everything was very complicated because at his deathbed Curt, was being treated differently from what he had expressed to her. Because she was "just his girlfriend" his children said she had no say in his treatment, and she was quickly outvoted. Because Curt had not written any of his wishes down or expressed them to his children, he died the way his children thought was best.

We need to clean up our own house. It is a very difficult subject to address for most of us, whether we are facing death or just randomly waiting our turn. There is a wonderful line from a television commercial that says it all: "Life's messy, clean it up!"

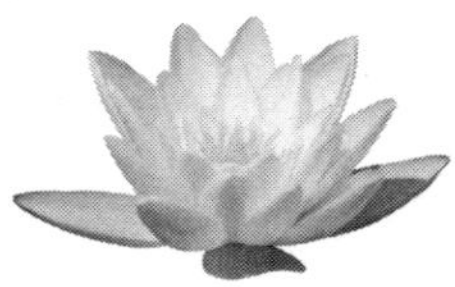

HEALERS: Healers are different from doctors. I do not consider doctors to be healers. They are too obsessed with curing. I have a simple way of dividing the two. Doctors need hospitals, machines, drugs and many years to work their magic. Healers perform under an elementary code of "Keep it simple, Sweetie!".

I went to a healer soon after my return from the Livingston Center. My friend Ann, gave me a gift of three visits to a "hands-on" healer. I was lucky that day because the healer had a woman apprentice with him. "A double whammy," I thought. The healers talked while they laid their hands in different areas of my body. I told them I recently had surgery for a cancerous tumor.

That was the extent I shared of my health history.

While lying on the table I experienced an increase of heat from their hands, but nothing exceptional. My real problem was my kidneys. I had been dealing with a kidney infection since my surgery and the chemotherapy. I did not mention this problem to either one of them. They did not ask; I did not tell. At the end of a 30 minute session, while putting my shoes on, the healer said, "We worked on your kidney infection. By tomorrow, it should be better." Somewhat skeptical, I said something like, "Oh...okay". While I was leaving, I hoped Ann had not spent a lot of money on this little gathering.

During the 50 mile drive home I had to stop and find a bathroom twice. I also began to sweat profusely, and my lower back was saturated with moisture through my clothes. That evening I continued to sweat until the next morning. I awoke feeling refreshed and amazingly well. I used up my two other gift certificates and paid for two more sessions on my own.

If you are skeptical about "healers", that is understandable. Unless you are Native American, most of us in this country have never seen a true healer in action. Most people are not believers, and would rather go to a doctor who will write out a prescription for their aches and pains.

Prayer healing is probably the most common and accepted form of hands-on healing. Many people gather around the sick person, putting their hands on the person and joining in prayer.

There is also psychic healing. A psychic healer talks to the sick person on the phone, holds a letter written by that person, or just images the person in their mind.

The types of healers are endless. I hope at one point in your healing experience that you engage the services of a healer. If anything, it will give you a new experience, a new awareness, a possible miracle. Albert Einstein once said, "There are two ways to live your life. One is as though nothing is a miracle. The other is as though everything is a miracle." Today, celebrate the miracle!

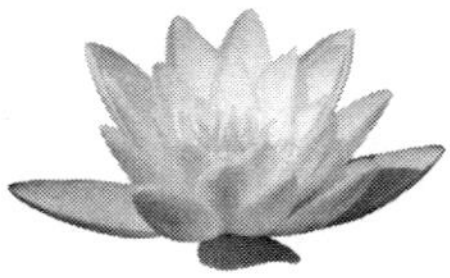

SPIRITUAL: Whether or not you believe in God is your business. Religion is one of the biggest complaints from the people who call me. A large majority told me they were already religious and had a belief in God. Their dissatisfaction came from other people assuming, "since this person is sick and has this dreadful disease, I have the right to enforce my personal beliefs."

I heard stories of this violation; things turned ugly; relationships went sour.

Whether or not you use the spiritual spoke is your choice. Just remember, being spiritual is a large category. Being spiritual is not only being religious, sacred... it is also, your mood and your attitude.

Prayer and chanting are simple spiritual endeavors. Or maybe you need to be in a large church with the pipe organ playing and moving your inner soul. For some people like myself, it's just me, my dogs and the trees and hills and wild animals created by someone more forgiving and loving than I.

A man named Simon told me his about his plight with cancer. He had a rare bone cancer in one leg. He had two tumors removed and was trying to prepare for the possibility of amputation. It was Sunday and Simon mentioned that he should be in church. "Then why aren't you?" I asked.

"I'm very angry at God. I'm Catholic and have gone to church my whole life. I feel betrayed." Simon told his plans to become an atheist. He had burned his rosaries, his medals and disposed of his statues. God was out of his life. I never felt drawn into this conversation; I only listened.

The next time Simon called me, he had made plans to travel. Simon worked for an airline which gave him the perfect opportunity to take off inexpensively.

The amputation of Simon's leg was scheduled in three weeks. His doctor did not see a problem with him taking this trip. It was over two months when I next heard from Simon. He was back at home packing his belongings. "Where are you headed now? And what about your leg? How did that work out?" I asked, not able to speak fast enough.

"You won't believe it, I found God again!" Simon sounded elated. "I traveled to France and ended up in Lourdes. I was only going to stay a couple of days, but I was drawn to the place and just couldn't leave. I stayed there for the whole three weeks. I met some people that volunteer to help the crippled and weak that can't make the walk. I was so consumed and forgot my own pain and agony. Everyday I witnessed many miracles. My leg appeared to have gotten worse. It was quite swollen and painful, but when I worked with the people who needed help each day, I forgot about everything."

After the three weeks, Simon knew he had to leave and face up to what was inevitable - the amputation of his right leg. He said he was given a special blessing before he left and a 50 person hands-on healing.

Prepared for the worst, he arrived at his doctor's office one week later. Simon was scheduled for surgery the following day, and took pre-op tests, including a CT scan. You have probably already guessed the ending. There was no longer the tube-size tumor alongside his leg bone. The doctor told Simon his cancer was in remission. Simon blurted out, "Remission, hell! It's a miracle, let's tell it like it is!"

Simon moved to Lourdes, France and is still witnessing miracles on a daily basis.

Physical things are weakened by the daily bombardment of the environment and continuous use. Mental and spiritual things are weakened by the absence of those shocks. Remaining mentally and spiritually powerful will help you emerge strengthened and even encouraged!

HUMOR: Norman Cousins told us many years ago about his discovery of the importance of humor and laughter in healing. Each week newspapers and magazines claim humor promotes healing. Then why are we not laughing? How long has it been since you had a good belly laugh? A laugh that made your stomach actually hurt, a fall-down-on-the-ground kind of laugh, one that brought real tears to your eyes?

In most of our daily lives we have to invent something to laugh about. Well, there is nothing wrong with that - invent away !

On your spoke you should have several ways to promote your daily laugh attacks. I cut out a photo of a dog from a local Pet Rescue newsletter and have it on my bathroom mirror. The dog is standing on his hind legs, front paws balanced against a chain link fence. His face is in an actual smile, tongue hanging out. Pure, raw, uncensored delight! I look at the photo every time I wash my face or brush my teeth. It always makes me laugh, no matter how many times I have seen it.

Like your daily vitamins and minerals which have a "recommended daily allowance", so should you have an RDA for laughter!

SANCTUARIES: Like humor, creating sanctuaries for yourself may be effective in your healing. People have told me about their favorite walking trails, beaches, forests, churches, animal preserves, and even libraries. Create many different sanctuaries for yourself. One may be hampered by the weather, or other people invading your favorite spot. Don't limit yourself. The pursuit of sanctuaries can be as healing as finding one. You can still have your favorite sanctuary, but always be on the lookout for others.

A woman named Carla lives in New Mexico. Her backyard

opens up to a large desert area where she can walk for miles without seeing another person. There are certain times of the year where she can not walk freely through the desert, because of the possibility of flash flooding. Carla was frustrated at first, until one day she looked out her kitchen window and spotted a rusted junk car her neighbor had left at the edge of their property line. She had seen that car for years and always hated the sight of it. That day outside of her kitchen window she saw it in a different light. It called to her. When she entered the backseat area where a door used to be, she knew she had found a new space for herself.

Even after years of neglect and exposure to the elements, the old leather seats were usable. The car was so old it had glass-stemmed vases hanging near the back windows. She discovered it had been a limousine for Hollywood celebrities in the 1930's.

Carla found her perfect sanctuary for the days she could not walk through the desert. She sat in her limousine and let her mind carry her to who might have sat on those same leather seats. At this writing, Carla is still dealing alternatively with her breast cancer, and still using her limousine. Her neighbor moved the vehicle closer to Carla's house and built a shelter around it.

Rodney called me after his last round of radiation for his

prostrate cancer. He was 32 years old with an incredible zest for life. He was seeking alternative treatments and preferred centers in foreign countries.

"I love finding new sanctuaries. I may never return to them, but I know what they look like and I can return anytime in my mind." I could hear Rodney drift away as he spoke. "I've got a big map of the world, and when I feel a bit down, or need to think things through, I look at the map and recall every sanctuary I have ever seen. I pick one, and I'm there, in my mind."

Instead of collecting antiques, coins or ceramic plates, collect sanctuaries. They're free, they're healing, and you will feel as rich as a land baron!

CELEBRATIONS: Most Americans celebrate Christmas, Thanksgiving or Fourth of July. Up to a certain age we celebrate birthdays. We are usually joyful at weddings, graduations and new babies. How many of us celebrate Wednesdays? Or three o'clock in the afternoon? Or like a friend told me, "just getting up!".

With our daily grind, it gets harder and harder to remember our personal celebrations. We are reminded of the larger, more obvious ones, because they are on calendars and most of the people we know are sharing that same celebration.

Like the spokes for HUMOR and SANCTUARIES, we need to create our own celebrations and hold to them. If someone is lacking self-esteem, they are just not celebrating life enough! With cancer, celebrations should be daily. Consider areas of treatment, marking the days, or by-passing doctor-imposed deadlines of your demise. Celebrations should reflect your life. They should show your accomplishments, your vitality, enthusiasm, compassion, your idealism - YOUR HEALING !

A couple of years ago David and I attended an Anthony Robbins seminar and we did a "firewalk". David and I had different reasons for celebrating this way. What an incredible commemoration! To walk on coals over 1200 degrees F. and not get burned, was certainly a celebration of the power of our minds! In Fiji the firewalk is used as a powerful healing ceremony. I do not suggest that you create your own firewalk with charcoal briquettes. Make sure you are dealing with someone like Tony Robbins who knows how to guide you through this experience.

Create grand celebrations and peaceful ones too. When we have many diverse celebrations our "possibility list" grows. We view the world with encouragement and joy!

When you are alone, REFOCUS YOUR THOUGHTS. Align with great ideas to use when fear returns. Stop analyzing. Give yourself some downtime. THIS IS WHERE COURAGE IS BORN!

CHAPTER NINE

When someone gets a disease, they become "born again" eaters. Mostly vegetarian.

What food do you daily "feed" your mind? Your mind is assaulted with negative, frightening thoughts, especially with a life-threatening disease. Now is the time to make your thoughts work for you ! Refocus your thinking. How do you do that? Make a list of positive thoughts, or thoughts that require some strategy, anything to pull you out of a downhill spiral.

Some people think they must analyze their cancer all of the time. Not so. When do you rest? When do you have a life? Constant grief has a physical affect on the body and causes loss of energy. You need that energy to function and heal. Set a time in the day that you work on or discuss your cancer. Then give yourself a break for the rest of the day.

At the Livingston Center I was busy each day, "working" on the cancer. By the second week, that time had diminished. When I left the Center for the day, the majority of my time was spent doing "normal" things.

Our mind can create its own atmosphere. It can store up the bright moments in our life, and use them as reserve power when we are experiencing sorrow or disappointment.

In 1969 during the height of the Vietnam War, I went to work for a civilian airline that was contracted with the United States government. We transported troops to and from Vietnam, part of the Military Air Command (MACV). My illustrious title was Flight Attendant. Six women on board a stretch DC-8 served 254 men and an occasional female nurse.

Those 254 men were comprised of four airline crew members and 250 military officers, medics, and draftees. In this sea of blue, khaki and green, it was difficult to experience anyone individually.

The work was hard, the hours were long and the war was treacherous. After three years at this job, I quit and withdrew to lick my wounds. I learned many facts of life on those flights. I learned war is serious business and did not resemble the John Wayne version. I learned how to refocus my thoughts. How to take myself out of a bad situation by changing my atmosphere and recalling my reserve power - those brighter moments of my life. Years later I realized how often I had done this refocusing.

The only smart thing I did during those crazy three years was to keep a journal. Reviewing the journal, years later, I saw a pattern in dealing with my problems and some of the bizarre experiences of the war. I was using my escape technique. It helped me, so I applied it.

As in my experience with cancer, my Vietnam encounter was riddled with stories of people beating the odds - heroes, creeps and violence. Somewhere between the creeps and the violence, I do remember losing my heart - my compassion. War and compassion mix like fire and wood. One consumes the other, leaving few traces of a previous life.

On one flight back to the States from Vietnam, I felt particularly agitated. We had been in Bien Hoa, Vietnam for three days. I felt like I was melting. The temperature was well over 100 degrees, the humidity the same. Our aircraft was set to go for two hours, but there was a hangup with the military protocol.

Someone had to stand at the bottom of each ramp, forward and aft, to greet the soldiers as they entered the aircraft. The six of us flipped for it, two of us lost. I positioned myself on the shady side of the ramp, but the tarmac boiled under my one inch regulation pumps.

I attempted to "remove" myself from this setting, but I had to keep one eye on the gate in case our passengers were unleashed. A big guy, stood first in line behind the gate. He was quite entertaining, and dressed in camouflage and heavy boots, jumping up and down and waving his process papers. Standing 100 feet away, I could see the biggest smile on any face in Southeast Asia. "Who is this nut?" I thought to myself.

All of the crew members had noticed him. Our senior flight attendant told us to keep an eye on him; she thought he had been drinking. I did not think so. It had been a long time since I saw this kind of behavior, but if you defined joy, we had witnessed it right before our eyes.

When the gate finally opened, Andy barreled out of it like a rodeo steer. He spoke in an Alabama drawl, but it was the fastest drawl I had ever heard. So fast, he spit as he talked. He kissed my hand, kissed the bottom step of the ramp and lumbered into the cabin of the aircraft.

Andy chose his seat like it had his name on it. He picked the seat next to the window by a wing exit and behind my jump-seat for landings and take-offs.

Preparing for take-off I took my seat in front of Andy. I noticed he was sitting with four shoe boxes tied together on his lap. Regulations required that all carry on luggage be put under the seat or in the overhead rack. I suggested that I needed to take his boxes and store them temporarily. He protested. By then the plane was in line for take-off. I broke regulation and let him keep his boxes on his lap.

I looked back at him one more time as the aircraft accelerated down the runway. He looked at me, smiled and as soft as this big guy could possibly speak, he said, "I'm goin' home." No one could have uttered those words more sincerely than Andy.

Throughout the flight, Andy entertained the whole crew and many of the men on the aircraft. What was so different was his innocence even after 13 months of combat. He talked about the letters he got from home and gestured to the 4 shoe boxes he held in his lap.

Home was a small town in Alabama. 250 people in the town, to be exact, and every one of them wrote to Andy while he was in Vietnam. They told him not to be a hero, but to stay alive and come back with all of his teeth in place. Andy said it was difficult at times and often he became discouraged, but he managed. Mainly because 250 people believed he could do it.

During the entire flight, Andy never budged from his seat. He said his uncle was the only one in his family who ever flew in an airplane before he left for Vietnam. His uncle told him where to sit and to "stay put." Andy sat with his boxes of letters, occasionally coaxed to read one more letter. None of us laughed at Andy. We experienced a brief moment of light in a dark period of our lives. I looked at the smiling faces surrounding Andy. Many had terrible encounters in Vietnam that would never leave them. Many had the worst of times still ahead of them. For that moment, time was suspended. Andy was our savior. He never knew how important he was in each of our lives.

I thought of the people that loved Andy, a whole town in Alabama. Somehow Andy was drafted. Those people in his town had to let him go, but they made sure they supported him and they kept him alive by sheer belief. They wrote Andy about the happenings on the farm. How the crops were growing and how many cows had new babies. Andy said most of the time he could forget about where he was and the letters took him home.

When the wheels of the aircraft touched the runway of Travis Air Force Base in California, the usual cheering took place. Except for Andy. I looked toward his seat and he had pressed his big face against the window. Tears streamed down his face and he did not try to cover them up. He said in a soft voice, "I'm home. I'm home." I believed him.

We all have two pairs of eyes. One pair is on our face, the other is in our mind. Most of us use only the eyes on our face. The mental eyes correct the errors of the physical eyes. They show brightness when physical eyes see only clouds.

When you are alone, "see" from your mind's eye. Change your scenery, get caught up in the brightness, not the cloud.

If asked about my ability to refocus my mind, I give the credit to the many POW's I met during my time in Vietnam. These courageous and determined men told me stories of how they lived through torture and confinement, as prisoners of war, for four, five, seven years!

One day I sat with a POW named Larry. I asked him how he was able to spend 5 years in confinement, never knowing from day to day if that would be his last moment on earth. Did he think we all abandoned him? And how about his family? His children were young when he last saw them. How did he feel about missing their prime growing years?

When I asked Larry, "How could your mind endure all of this?" he opened up.

"It wasn't that bad. I kept busy everyday. In the morning, I played a round of golf, in the afternoon I practiced and played my guitar, and in the evening I played in a small band."

"Wow, that's amazing!" I said naively "I didn't know you had such luxuries."

"We didn't. I did all of that stuff in my mind!"

Larry "played" golf every day in his mind and got so good that he could lose himself in his "game" for 3 to 4 hours a day. After he rested, he "practiced" his guitar. This occupied 2 to 3 hours a day. Later in the evening, Larry imaged himself "jamming" with some friends at a local pub near his house back in the States.

When Larry returned home, he enjoyed golf regularly with a 3 handicap. He practiced his guitar and jammed on weekends with his buddies at the local pub.

Larry had many difficulties to overcome, but he continued to use his mind technique upon returning to his former life. Larry knew, in order to make sure that those years spent as a POW were not in vain, he had to continue to live his life as best he could. Being captured by the Viet Cong, enduring torture and confinement were not Larry's original goal. This was his fate, his destiny and he was wise enough to make good use of whatever was served to him.

I learned a lot from people like Larry. When the moment came for me to step up to the plate, I recalled the many stories I had heard and developed my own mind technique. Lying in my hospital bed, after my cancerous tumor was removed, I used my mind to "change my atmosphere." It was now my turn to find my courage and get on with life, though it was not what I had planned.

When my fear was so bad, so awful that my hands were shaking, I made myself "walk" the path I had walked everyday at home. I made myself "smell" the air, "listen" for the quail, "feel" my feet on the granite rocks smattered with pine needles and leaves.

I concentrated on my "surroundings," bringing myself back to the trees I loved so much. I looked for branches that I could take home with me to "carve". My hunt brought me back to my studio where I "felt" the mallet and carving tools I used to create my humorous sculptures.

When I became real good at my mind technique, I started "carving" in my mind. I could "hear" the mallet hit the end of the carving tool and saw the wood chips flying off of the piece. I lost myself in this process!

I "created" a cocky alligator on a motorcycle that "rode" up the hospital stairway, did a wheelie in my room and took me away from the madness, hospital-gown and all!

I "carved" a six foot rabbit, dressed him in a white dinner jacket and gave him a silver tray to hold. I thought he could help me during my recovery. What a stupendous time I had - me, myself and I, and of course all of the "animals" I "created" in my mind!

When I did return to work I actually created those same animals in real life! It was an incredible Zen experience. My hands worked like they were preprogrammed!

For those first few months after my surgery, when the fear returned or I had to deal with the insensitivities of some people, I questioned the path of my recovery. Several times a day I forced myself to use my mind technique. I became a very prolific artist!

Soon my mind understood the association; fear equals carved animal. It has now become automatic, I no longer have to force myself to do this. No matter where I am, in a crowd of people or alone, I "carve" animals shamelessly. I first create my sculptures by imaging them in my mind. Then I find the wood and lastly, I physically carve the piece.

I believe this mind technique can be life saving. It can be used in many areas of your life, but it has to be used consistently. In our world of instant gratification, people have condemned its practice because it requires persistence and COURAGE! Why courage? Because people do not make full use of their brain-power. When you are using your brain-power - worry and doubt tag along for the ride. At first they will be everpresent, but if you persist with your mind technique they will soon leave you. Once you have conquered your anxiety, what will be revealed is a sense of power to make yourself strong. You must use it as a habit and not as an occasional calling of effort.

People are fascinated by my use of this mind technique. When

I speak publicly about it, I bring along the art pieces I created in my mind while lying in the hospital. I receive many questions and generate a lot of interest in my mind technique. The sad fact is that most of the interest dies out the very first day. Or I receive questions several days following my talk. "Is there an easier way?"

Plain and simply, NO. By assuming the habit of calling on your brain-power you are promoting action, and the more you call upon that power, the stronger it will grow and the greater will be your success.

I have had a life filled with risk-taking events that took courage. The most courageous action was sitting across from my oncologist after he had just explained the necessity of doing at least one year of chemotherapy or accepting an early death, and I said NO. I said NO to what was accepted in treating cancer. I said No to my fear and YES to a small spark I felt gaining ground inside me.

I did not walk away without a plan. I had an idea where I was going, but it was all new territory for me. My legs shook as I walked out of my oncologist's office, but by the time I had reached my car I had "carved" a frog playing a piano. In my mind the frog's piano tunes drown the sound of my doctor's words.

If you have been timid in the past, for goodness sake, take your courage in both hands and make full use of your brain-power!

Cancer promotes change. START YOUR TRANSFORMATION NOW.

CHAPTER TEN

Human nature is slow to change. Many of us stay in a situation that offers grief and still we make no effort to change. Until the pain of change is less painful then the situation, we remain in our quagmire.

A life threatening disease is enough for people to change. For some, the transformation is slow and progressive. For others, it is overnight. It does not always depend on the severity of the disease.

I have talked with people who are told they are terminal, stage 4. Some of them chose not to change any part of their lives until they saw their lives failing. Then change came quickly, sometimes not quickly enough.

Start your transformation now. How radical you change is up to you. These 15 decisions applied will move you in a new direction. These 15 decisions have been tried and recommended by over five hundred people who have walked the same path ahead of you. Call on their experience. You will see and feel more control over your disease.

Everyone I interviewed about cancer had a story to tell about their eventual change. One woman named Luanne created the biggest transformation from the most benign beginning. Luanne said she had cancer of the cervix. She left me a long, drawn-out, hysterical message on my answering machine. When I connected with Luanne she was still hysterical and crying uncontrollably. The first two calls were cut short because she could not contain herself enough to converse.

Three weeks had passed before Luanne made her third attempt to talk with me. She had not made any decisions on her course of action concerning her cancer.

"What are your doctor's suggestions for treatment?" I asked.

"I don't know," she replied. "How progressive does he think your cancer is?" "I don't know," she repeated.

I was at a loss for words. For someone who was so hysterical about her news to not know the extent of her disease, just didn't fit. People like Luanne normally know everything about their disease. Often their hysteria comes from knowing too much medical terminology and feeling overwhelmed and out of control by their knowledge.

The next time Luanne left a frantic message on my answering machine, I didn't call her until later that evening. I was hoping she would collect her emotions and be able to talk. She sounded much better when she answered the telephone. She told me she called her doctor and told him she wanted to discuss his suggestions for her treatment. It had been almost a month since she last saw him and she felt she was strong enough to face what was before her. When Luanne went to her doctor's office and was sitting across from him, she felt her emotions well up once more. He was trying to tell Luanne what he would recommend when she got up and ran out of his office.

"Luanne, you know you can't continue to run away from this. You have many options, but we can't discuss them until we know just what you are dealing with."

"I know, I know," she cried, "I always end up dealing with everything in my life this way. I've run away from people, jobs, everything...this is no exception. I will call my doctor back tomorrow and discuss his prognosis, I promise. I'll call you back."

I felt confident that Luanne had finally reached her peak of hysteria and could now deal with what she had to confront. Two weeks passed before I made another call to her.

Luanne answered the telephone and sounded entirely different. Her voice was sing-song and she sounded happier. She apologized for not getting back to me sooner. She said she did return to her doctor's office, but this time she was armed with copies of articles she researched on cervical cancer and the use of radiation and chemotherapy as treatments. Her research showed poor results from both treatments.

Luanne went on for another ten minutes discussing the research she had discovered. I interrupted her by asking, "What is the extent of your cancer and have you decided to have surgery and what kinds of treatment will you follow up with?"

Still in her sing-song voice, Luanne said, " I won't be having surgery or any follow up treatments, for that matter. When I finally did listen to my doctor I found out I had jumped the gun a bit. I don't have cervical cancer, I have a precancerous condition of the cervix. It seems I just heard the word "cancerous" and I was off and running. Hello... are you still there, Micki?"

Slowly I regained my composure. "Do you do this "off and running" stuff frequently?"

"Yes, I admit, I have been accused of doing this before," Luanne giggled, "but a precancerous condition is like a time bomb ready to go off, I..." I cut her off. "Before I hang up and get back to my life I want you to know that I agree with you that a precancerous condition <u>can</u> be serious. Did you know that if you have any moles, or sometimes called "beauty marks," that those also are precancerous? I never try to judge people, Luanne, or condemn someone for how they handle bad news in their lives, but I am going to make an exception with you. You are a wimpy woman! Your overreaction and hysteria is an embarrassment to me, and the hundreds of women I have talked with, who have handled their more severe situations with dignity. You still could not find the courage to even let me know your findings. Instead you chose to let me simmer and worry about you. Grow up, not everything is about you!"

I was outraged. My time and energy and telephone bills were wasted on a self-centered, little girl who made me reconsider why I was continuing to talk with people about their options.

Two months later, I received a long letter from Luanne. She began by apologizing and then went into the changes she had made since our conversation. She had lived in a house she inherited from her parents and lived off of her inheritance. She sold her house and started a Foundation for low income women to get medical testing and treatments. Luanne bought a building that was converted into a medical center. She now lives in a small apartment in the rear of the building. She is on call 24 hours a day to help women and their children.

Luanne wrote in her letter that her plans were to do this for two years in hopes that the courage of these other women would "rub off on her."

She continues to write and call me. She has had her up and down periods, but she is finding courage within herself.

When we are told we have a life threatening disease, something changes within us. It is not the same for each person, but for some, their whole being is different. Our lives, or parts of it, become square pegs trying to fit back into round holes. Even if we are healed, going back to our same lives is not possible.

My own transformation took on many forms. In some areas I moved slower, in others it was overnight. My biggest transformation came in the way of understanding we have many choices, many options, in everything we do. The people who call me think there is only one way to treat cancer. I thought that once. I even believed that my misfortune of not having health insurance would be the death of me. It was not, but I lived for years feeling I was cheated by the circumstance that caused my inability to obtain health insurance.

While I was working as a Flight Attendant in Vietnam, I was exposed to the herbicide Agent Orange. When I got very ill on one flight, I was sent to the company doctor. Tests were done which showed an irritation on my skin which caused my skin to swell, ooze and peel. I ran a high temperature for several days and felt flu-like symptoms. This skin "rash" was mostly on my face. I was put on leave for over two months until the condition subsided and went away. Everytime I became stressed the condition flared up again. When I left the company, I was notified that I had what might be an exposure to the defoliants used in Vietnam.

While in Vietnam I drank out of open barrels of water while watching the helicopters release the last of their canisters marked with an orange stripe, commonly called Agent Orange. There was also Agent white, red, blue and DDT.

Prior to my leaving the airline, I received a notice from my insurance company stating I had "chloracne". The next time I applied for health insurance after my airline insurance ran out, I was denied. I tried again, I was denied. An insurance agent who investigated my denial found the computer to say it was "war related". For years I fought this injustice. I also found out that "chloracne" is a result of Agent Orange. The fact that I was a civilian in Vietnam gave me very little recourse. Until the day I found out I had cancer, I had agonized over my health insurance dilemma.

When I heard the news of the cancer, one of the worst insurance nightmares turned out to be a "little man with a large bullhorn".

At first it is not easy to live in our society without the protection of health insurance. Soon, you discover another world. A very big and exciting world of CHOICES! You need to move into this world a transformation of your thinking, a paradigm shift, and the courage to make that move. In this big, alternative world, there are still structures of conventional medicine practices. You will not enter a new dimension, just a new paradigm.

Personal transformation starts with personal responsibility for our own lives. There is punishment for shirking our responsibility. It lies in appearing inconsistent in our powers of mind and body. The reward lies however, in accepting our responsibilities, in the glory of achievement and the pleasure of discovering new and unsuspected powers.

Although the snake will never win a favorite pet award, many people acknowledge its ability to change form and survive the test of time. Once you recognize the power of transformation you will never return to your old skin again.

Make yourself LAUGH BEFORE YOU CRY.

CHAPTER ELEVEN

"There is nothing wrong with the salty taste of tears," said my friend Jack. " I just prefer the ache in my stomach from laughter." He wasn't kidding. Jack laughed more than any person I ever met. It was a giggle followed by a snort, or excess saliva sprayed in all directions. Or the loss of his glasses, or even his footing. Jack had fun. The fifteen years I knew Jack were full of laughter. The few times we had misunderstandings, he could not stay serious for more than five minutes. The corners of his mouth would be straining to break into a smile. It was hopeless to be serious with Jack.

Jack was 25 years older than me and a great friend. He had an airplane. I was taking flying lessons, so we teamed up and had a ball. Jack had financial difficulties, a wife with health problems, and personal obstacles like being in a wheel chair. Jack laughed his way through it all. He was born happy.

Jack died of a massive stroke. Before he died he left a message on my answering machine. He told a joke. The joke was less than a minute, but his laughter was five minutes. I could hear his glasses fall. He laughed uncontrollably, snorted and for a few seconds I thought he had stopped breathing. Of course I did not remember the joke, just Jack's laughter. I still remember it when I know I am letting my life get far too serious.

Jack died at age 69. His laughter did not extend his life beyond the norm, but it may have added years. Jack had serious medical problems for over twenty years. When doctors looked at CT scans of his brain, Jack was told that he should not be alive. Jack just laughed.

Scientists have studied laughter and why some people are happier than others. Findings show that 50% of happiness comes from birth, the other 50% is learned. It comes from our outlook in life and how we deal with the cards we are dealt.

The now deceased author, Norman Cousins, became well-known for his book, *ANATOMY OF AN ILLNESS* . He believed he was able to help his healing experience through laughter. Since Norman Cousin's book, many other people have come to the same conclusion - that laughter contributed to their healing.

I am very lucky to have known people like my friend Jack, who laughed through life or used humor as a mainstay. They were good role models when I was challenged with life's pressing problems.

Dan called me one day to tell me of his prostate cancer. He seemed to be an agreeable chap until we talked about laughing before you cry.

"I'm dying, what's so funny about that?" Dan grumbled. We discussed the fact that his dying was not funny, it was the stuff surrounding the circumstance that was humorous. "Like what?" Dan asked.

"I don't know, think about it. Was there an incident that took place in your treatments that you found even a bit funny?" I was beginning to think about changing the subject.

"You mean like the time I was waiting to get the results of a test and I'm sitting in a waiting room. My bladder's filled with three quarts of water and I'm ready to burst, but they don't want me to relieve myself 'cause I may have to do the test over again, and I say 'Hell with them' and walk over to the potted plant and my bladder's thanking me six ways to Sunday?" Dan and I both laughed so hard we could not speak for a minute or so until he started again.

"Or the time my doctor, who's a young, dapper fella and very serious, bends over to pick up his prescription pad and farts a big one, and me and the nurse bust out laughin'?" More laughter. "Or the time I returned to the same waiting room to take another test and found the infamous potted plant was gone! And my wife was with me and I told her what I did and she had to leave the room 'cause we were laughing so much?"

When I regained my composure, I said, "I think you got it Dan. Yeah, I think you could teach it!" Dan started in again, "Or the time..."

A hearty chuckle is your body's best antidote for anxiety. A big belly laugh stretches the muscles from the diaphragm to your scalp, releasing tension and all that comes with it. Laughter also boosts circulation and oxygen in the blood, giving you a burst of energy. Some researchers suggest that laughing releases endorphins, the body's natural painkillers and mood elevators.

Some people take naps. You might want to take a laugh break. This will take some doing at first, but like Dan you will be able to store up those memories and recall them anytime.

Nine months after my surgery and diagnosis of cancer, I decided what our town needed was a community event. I live in the heart of the Napa Valley in California, the main growing region of premium California wines. Every October we have an annual Harvest Festival. It is a community event that people attend after the rush of the harvest. The Festival needed a shot in the arm. Attendance was trailing and we needed something that would kick the day off with laughter. What better way to get this agricultural community together than with a Pet Parade? People here love their animals. David and I organized the parade to benefit our local animal society. We put up our own money to get the parade idea rolling and we expected a modest crowd. We struck a nerve, the humorous nerve to be exact. That first year we had 125 participants and hundreds of people lined the streets! Now the Pet Parade is an anticipated event and grows larger each year.

What the town doesn't know is that each year when they come to enjoy and laugh at the Pet Parade, they are helping me celebrate another year of being healed! I can not imagine celebrating any better than with people who have supported me, animals and laughter!

Laugh, my friend, laugh!

Fill your hospital room or home with FUN, WHIMSICAL ART or pictures from a magazine of places where your mind can go when you need strength.

CHAPTER TWELVE

Our bodies and minds respond to beauty, of form, of scent, or of sound. Our bodies and minds respond to humor, magnificence and colors. It amazes me why hospitals use the same tired decor. Many have decorated their lobbies and waiting rooms, but how about the patient's rooms?

I asked a hospital administrator why they couldn't spiff up the patient's rooms and her reply was, "The patients are so sick they don't really care." Oh really? I thought back to my hospital stay on the cancer ward. David and my family decorated my room with my art and pictures and sayings on the walls. Everyday I had visitors from all over the ward, other cancer patients and staff, just to see the art. A lot of these people were very sick, but they heard there was someone on the ward who had something else to look at besides a television and an institutional green wall.

Art speaks volumes. It was the earliest form of writing, when our ancestors conveyed meaning to one another through crude pictures. In one sculptural form or a square canvas, an artist can convey a story or a thought. A writer can only impart meaning through hundreds of words.

I have artist friends who create humorous art. We have had conversations about doing art for hospitals and "quiet rooms." Each one of us have been asked to submit ideas for similar projects. Each one of us have been turned down. "Too silly." "Not serious enough." "Too out there." "That would be great for the children's ward, but not for adults."

Since hospitals are businesses they should offer people a choice, and not assume that people do not care. I care, and I know many other people do also. Especially since the overnight room rate is so high. Imagine going to a hospital and being asked to choose from several different room categories? Maybe the Monet room, the Salvador Dali room, or the George Rodrique and his Blue Dog room. Or other artists like cartoonist Gary Larson, Picasso, Red Grooms. I realize that original art from well-known artists is expensive, but there are many local artists in any area that can be paid to integrate their work into a hospital setting.

For some people, their hospital room is the last place they will spend time before they die. Art is not only seen with our eyes, we feel it.

If hospitals choose to ignore the healing power of art, it does not mean you cannot add what you appreciate. This can be part of your transformation. If you cannot afford original art, then have someone shop local art festivals or cut out pictures from magazines.

As an artist I am amazed how often I hear people say they do not have an imagination. I tell them, that is their imagination! They have imaged no imagination. Art eludes many people.

A woman named Dorothy talked to me about her recovery from cancer surgery. She was at home and bored with television and felt she was in too much pain to read. I suggested she explore art that she liked and also art that was challenging.

"I don't know anything about art or what kind of art I would really like," she grumbled.

I recommended that she start by looking through magazines. Dorothy had her husband bring some. She particularly liked the Southwest Art magazine, because she was originally from New Mexico. Dorothy called me often to tell me of her recovery progress and the new interest she and her husband discovered in art.

They fell in love with Southwest painters and sculptors and soon planned a trip to the Southwest, connecting the dots to the different locations of each artist they liked. I received a postcard from Dorothy on their trip. They had purchased several pieces of art and could not wait to live with them at their home. They thanked me for introducing them to "a most marvelous creation" - their imagination!

Do not let anyone tell you that you are in denial. YOU ARE IN REALITY!

CHAPTER THIRTEEN

How often have you had a conversation with someone about a friend and said "She's in denial?" Many of us have used that term. What I believe we are saying is that <u>we</u> do not understand them or the direction they have chosen. I have argued this point with therapist friends until we are both blue in the face. This is a very popular term in therapy. The rest of us are parroting it. It is also a popular term used with life threatening illnesses.

When I was first diagnosed with cancer, I learned that if I did not lay down and say "Do anything to me" that I was told I was in denial. Since the path I chose for treatment was not the conventional one, I was assaulted with the "you-are-in-denials," even by my doctor.

In Webster's dictionary, there are several definitions for "denial." "Refusal" or "to refuse" is consistently used with each definition. To refuse or to decline to accept or reject is called denial. I find that interesting, since I refused to accept what my doctor told me I needed to do for a treatment. Otherwise, he said I would die within a year. I also rejected the standard cancer treatments. Sounds like I was heavy in denial, but also still living!

I have talked with people who have rejected the idea that they have cancer, period. This drives therapist's crazy. I met two people who are still alive today who have refused to consider cancer as a life threatening illness. They both had to break away from family and friends because their thinking was so radical. These people are in their eighth and tenth cancer free years.

James is a man who thinks for himself. When he called to talk about his prostate cancer, we talked about the "denial theory."

"The way I see it," said James, "is that other people are <u>threatened</u> by my illness, I'm not." It must be true. James has already lived five years past the time his doctor told him his demise would occur. If James is "in denial," then that is where I want to be.

Some people are threatened by mental independence. With life threatening illnesses, we are not expected to understand this complex issue. We are expected to leave it to someone else more qualified. We have a tendency to get our thoughts from those whose credibility is a degree framed on a wall. When we turn our back on the accepted way, we are scorned and treated like children. When we decide for ourselves the right method for our healing, we make others who have set the standards uneasy and fearful.

There are people who cannot make a decision, even if their life depended on it. Those people would probably not be reading this book or even considering other options.

Most of the people I have interviewed were "living in denial" like James. They shared the belief that their minds were capable of solving their difficulties, even if that difficulty were death.

Karen spent most of our conversation discussing the fact that her family and friends were suggesting that she was in denial. Karen chose to skip chemotherapy for the Burzynski program in Houston, Texas. Her family did an "intervention" with her. They showed up at her house and tried to convince her of her mistake. She laughed, telling me about the graphs and charts her brother put together to help prove his point. Karen said they must said, "you're in denial" over thirty times! She listened and then asked if they had said all that they wanted to say. When no one had anything more to add, Karen took the floor.

"You are entitled to believe and accept what you want. If or when you are confronted with a disease, I hope you will listen and depend on the faculties of your own mind that will naturally rally to your assistance. Don't tell me that I am in denial. Take a long look at your own lives. I'm in reality!"

When friends told me they thought I was in denial when I chose to do alternative medicine, I could not help but look at their lives. Their relationships were disastrous; they had severe financial problems and their children were three steps from the doors of juvenile hall. There will always be people who will not understand and will be threatened by your decisions. Consider the following ideas:

1. Keep yourself focused and have several plans. Plan A, B, and C. You will have considered other options and have other choices to fall back on.
2. Listen to other advice, but think for yourself.
3. Embrace your fear. Let it make you stronger; it is a useful emotion.
4. Visualize your outcome in your treatments and discussions with family members.
5. Turn your weaknesses into strengths. Show your family and friends that you truly believe in what you are doing. When you are frightened let them know, but show your strength in reserving your right to do what you believe is the right path.

Never mind if people think you are wrong or foolish. Until they are in your shoes, they cannot judge. Let them think you are in denial. What does it matter? If you listen to other people and let yourself be guided only by them, you bind yourself by the limits of their minds, and unless, by some chance, those who are guiding you are large-minded, you will cramp your spirit and your intuition for your remaining days.

Using war terminology to describe a disease or how you are dealing with it is not healing. Diseases take time to heal and one cannot sustain a "battle" for long. SAY, "I AM HEALING!"

CHAPTER FOURTEEN

"Do I have to be a warrior?" asked thirteen year old Katy. She walked up to me after my speech. Katy had bone cancer. "What do you want to be?" I asked her. "I'd prefer to be an otter. They like to play and have fun. I'm not real sure what warriors do, but I know they're involved with fighting or something like that... since I already have cancer, I don't want more negative stuff in my life."

I could not agree more with Katy. When I hear someone use the term "war on cancer" or they talk about "battling cancer," my hackles go up. Maybe it comes from my experience in Vietnam during the war. I was not directly involved in the fighting, but I spent plenty of time in the bunkers and heard endless stories of battles.

In a battle there is a winner and a loser, or two losers. Usually the winner even comes out bloodied. Battles vary in length but most do not last long. There is an enemy and that enemy is portrayed as evil and domineering.

When I was diagnosed with cancer it was evident how much war terminology is used to describe the experience of a cancer patient. I heard the comparison a few times from my friends. Soon I stopped them in mid-sentence and told them, "I am not a cancer survivor. I am not surviving, I am thriving!"

Here is an example if we put it in terms of finances and you asked me, "How is your financial situation, Micki?" And I answered you by saying, "It's surviving." What picture comes to your mind about my financial situation? Rather grim, I suspect.

Turn it around and instead say, "my financial situation is thriving!" My finances could still be shaky, but that is a more positive and focused thought. Most importantly, I believe it!

People who have not had cancer are more likely to use this reference. When you are immersed in a life threatening disease you soon tire of this rhetoric. If someone is "battling" cancer, they cannot sustain that battle for too long. There is always an enemy in war. So I ask you, if you choose to think of the cancer as the enemy and it is in your body, doesn't that make your body the enemy also? How healing is that?

Some people say, "no, the cancer is the enemy." Go back and review history and actual wars of the past. In Vietnam, we identified the enemy as the Viet Cong. The entire country, the women and children and the environment were maimed, destroyed or killed along with many of the Viet Cong.

If someone feels they can better heal themselves and they are motivated by using war terminology, then who am I to tell them differently?

My suggestion though, would be to stop and listen to what you are saying and believing. If "we are what we think" and "what we believe, we can conceive" are true, then you get the picture.

Former President Richard Nixon declared the war on cancer

in the early 1970's. It was not appropriate then and it is not appropriate now.

You do not need to "battle" or "fight" or become a "warrior". There are many other empowering ways for you to think about the cancer. The word disease can be broken up and looked at as a dis-ease of the body. One woman told me she thought of her cancer like an ex-boyfriend. Always hanging around and calling until she took steps to eliminate him from her life. He continued to persist for awhile but soon lost interest in her.

If someone asks you, "how is your battle going?" say "I'm healing!" and leave it at that.

A positive attitude is very important.

BACK UP YOUR ATTITUDE WITH ACTION!

CHAPTER FIFTEEN

"You will need more than a positive attitude to cure yourself from your cancer," my oncologist said just before we hung up. He was right. A healthy and positive attitude is a good attribute when you are dealing with a life threatening disease. An attitude, though, is just an attitude, unless you back it up with action.

Summoning your fortitude, optimism and your faith is a great way to begin. Without the vibration of action to accompany your quest, you are vulnerable to the jaws of the big, bad wolf - DOUBT.

In the area of life threatening illnesses, every person needs to be a pioneer. Each one of us is so different, so individual. Why are we still being treated the same for cancer? You do not need to become the Great Explorer and go forth to the wastelands of alternative medicine. You can blaze your own little trail and still not be foolhardy. If you choose to stay within the confines of what your doctor and your insurance company have set for you and you are not healing, what will it take for you to take action and look in other directions?

Start by "window-shopping" or use the "just-looking" attitude. Call people who have the same cancer, but who did alternative treatments. Or they complimented their conventional treatment with alternative choices.

The Internet is a wealth of information. If you have the

capability to use the Net, you will be amazed what is available world-wide in treatments. The Internet is doing the most to promote change in our present health system. It is not censored. As a pioneer, you must research and read all that is available on a particular treatment. Because the Net is not censored, you will need to balance your skepticism and open-mindedness.

People have told me about their research on the Internet or otherwise. When they took the research to their doctors they were often scoffed and told that they were wasting their precious time. If there were a cure, their doctor would have known about it.

Janet took her research to her doctor. He laughed out loud. "You would be better off sticking to your positive attitude instead of wasting your time doing research. At least with a positive attitude, you'll get points in heaven. If there were anything out there that could save your life, I would know about it!"

Janet said she kept her cool, but informed her doctor that she would not be returning any more. She was a devout Catholic and decided to leave her doctor with an award winning speech. "Am I to give up because you fear my death? Can I suppose that the Being who placed me here, Who gave me the right to think and act for myself, Who filled the world with loveliness, music, and more, will blame me for assuming my rights, or will give me anything less bountiful in the world to come? It is against all logic and common sense and I will not believe it!"

Believe in yourself and your decisions.

YOU ARE RIGHT!

CHAPTER SIXTEEN

RISK! RISK ANYTHING! CARE NO MORE FOR THE OPINIONS OF OTHERS. DO THE HARDEST THING ON EARTH FOR YOU. ACT FOR YOURSELF. FACE THE TRUTH.

- KATHERINE MANSFIELD

There is a "magic bullet" to overcoming cancer. I know, I know - I am sticking my neck out by making such a statement. The "magic bullet" does not cost you one cent or falsely raise your hopes. This magic bullet is YOU!

You are the single greatest factor in preventing and overcoming cancer. Your own personal knowledge is one of your most powerful tools against a disease.

I suggest you learn about your particular cancer to empower yourself to make the choices you believe are the best for you. I encourage you to FOCUS NOT on the cancer but on YOUR HEALING. Reserve a time for researching your dis-ease, but do not make it your top priority. It is my experience that we receive what we focus on.

Consider my eight year old buddy, Elvis, from Oklahoma City. When Elvis' father, Cliff, called me three years ago, Elvis was five and struggling to stay alive. Elvis had bone cancer and had already endured six months of chemotherapy, hanging on to life by a thread.

Besides the misfortune of Elvis' fate, the compounding tragedy was that Elvis' mother had died two years before Elvis was diagnosed with bone cancer. She had the same disease.

Cliff and Elvis were very close and Cliff told me that his strength came from his small son. During a conversation with Cliff, I violated one of my own rules when I said "Elvis sounds like a brave young guy."

Cliff immediately replied, "No, he's not brave. He's not fighting a war, he's healing his body! We focus only on his healing!"

That sure put me in my place. Every conversation after that moment began with "How is Elvis healing?" Cliff would reply, "He tells me that he feels he's making progress."

During those first few conversations I honestly just played along because I thought it helped Cliff.

For two more months Elvis barely clung to life. One day I received a call from Cliff. I began with my usual, "How is Elvis healing?", expecting Cliff's usual reply. Instead Cliff said, "Why don't you ask him yourself? I'll put him on the phone."

I did ask Elvis. A weak but enthusiastic voice said, "I told my dad that I would be fine - you gotta focus on the good stuff ONLY!"

Once we began to doubt ourselves, this constant drip of our

"leaky faucet" is not easily repaired. Doubt has been the culprit of bringing down even the best and the brightest amongst us. Hundreds of people have become wealthy enlightening us about our doubts. When we learn how to control the doubt in one area of our lives, we find weakness in another. It could almost feel entirely hopeless, except for one truth. Doubt is always cloaked in appearances. Appearances are the food for doubt. Without the *thought of appearances*, doubt shrivels and starves to death.

If you look upon the appearance of disease, you will produce that form of disease in your own mind - and ultimately in your own body. Instead, you must *hold the thought of the truth*, which is *there is no disease*. Disease is only an appearance, ***the reality is health.***

It takes power *to think health* when surrounded by the appearance of disease, or surrounded by the promotion of hopelessness, anxiety, anger, and war related ideas. It requires power to trust that small voice within and ignore the chorus of outside voices. Even those voices of our families, doctors, well-meaning friends and the media.

To hold the *thought of truth* is truly the hardest work in the entire world. To learn to control your appearances, you must understand that every sustained thought becomes a form, and that form becomes visible. Once you learn this, you lose all doubt and fear because you know that you can create what you want to create.

This is your "magic bullet". It is YOU, YOUR THOUGHTS, YOUR FOCUS. I found my magic bullet. Many of the people in this book found their magic bullet along the way to healing. We did not know what we were looking for. We were anxious and fearful and even full of doubt. At a certain point in my healing, this became as evident as a highway billboard. To others it was a voice as tiny as a peeping baby chick. When you do hear it, take Katherine Mansfield's advice, "Risk! Risk anything! Care no more for the opinions of others. Do the hardest thing on earth for you. Act for yourself. Face the truth."

In dealing with cancer, our doubt is perpetuated by years and millions of people dying young or old from this horrifying disease. We hear that one out of three will get cancer in our lifetime and that cancer now ranks as the second most common cause of death after heart disease. Our doubts and fears are bestowed upon us each day by the media. With this daily bombardment of negative information, you must make a complete paradigm shift here or a complete transformation to keep doubt from consuming your life.

The people in this book and the hundreds of others I have interviewed, vote their physicians the biggest doubt caster!

When we walk into a doctor's office, who is the authority figure? We do not know medicine so we place our trust in the doctor.

One day I talked to a woman named Annie who was a dog trainer. Annie had breast cancer and was very frustrated with her doctor and his suggested treatment. She thought it would be a good idea for doctors to restore the policy of making house calls. That way they would be on your turf and as she said laughingly, "Less territorial!"

Annie might have the right idea. Being a dog trainer, she knows how dogs relate to a stranger when one comes to their house. If you bring most dogs to another house that they are not familiar with they will not act as the dominant one.

Until the practice of house calls is reinvented, learn to use your doctor as your consultant, not as your case manager. In truth, orthodox medicine does not provide a full spectrum of health care options. It has created a niche which is limited to surgery and pharmacology. How can a doctor who has a closed mind to everything but drugs and surgery, make the ideal decision for you? Are medications and having an operation, the only solution for you? Do you really believe that one health problem, has no relationship to any other health problem you have? Is your doctor so familiar with your life that he knows you will not be able to overcome a disease?

Only the body can heal itself. Your doctor cannot. Your doctor can consult, suggest, recommend and point you in some direction, but your body does all of the work. 98% of the atoms that make up your body were not there a year ago. That change had nothing to do with your doctor but had all to do with YOU. Avoid the obedient mediocrity. Believe in yourself and your decisions.

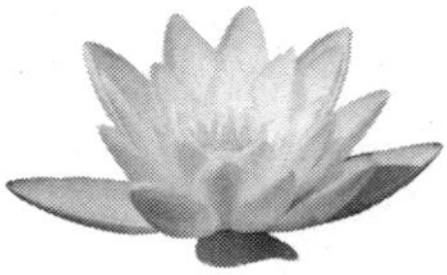

Elvis and his father were forced to stay within the law and were left with only the option of chemotherapy. But it was this little boy, namesake of the King of Rock and Roll, who understood what really controlled his healing.

For the next two years I continued to talk with Elvis and his dad, Elvis had three serious setbacks, and each time he was told by his doctors that he was in his "final days". Each time Elvis and Cliff focused "on the good stuff ONLY" and Elvis proved all of his doctors "full of the stuff that's between your toes".

During Elvis' third setback, I heard Cliff's voice falter for the first time. "I think this really might be our final round. I don't think Elvis is going to make it."

Ordinarily, I would have agreed, but Elvis was not ordinary. He was extraordinary. I knew Cliff was tired and *human*, but I reminded him of "focusing on the good stuff ONLY". Cliff was extraordinary too and soon regained his composure. He concluded with, "Elvis is right. We just need to believe in our personal healing."

Two weeks later I played a message on my answering machine and recognized Cliff's voice. He was in his car driving Elvis home from the hospital. Jokingly, he left this message, " ELVIS HAS LEFT THE BUILDING!"

Elvis has been in remission for over two years.

Treating cancer is your business. HEAL WITH IT!

CHAPTER SEVENTEEN

I am hoping you receive from this book, the understanding that what fuels the human spirit is not intellectual certainty, but things like belief, hope, love and the trust of your intuition to guide you to move in the right direction. You might say that the business that we are all in as humans is to gain insight of our spirit, or life force. Without that life force - well, we are just plain out of business. We have died.

When we have cancer, our "business" is to find what is left of our life force and restore it. In many ways, it might need a renovation, it might need to spend more time "being" and less time "doing". In any case, life force, or our spirit, is all that separates each of our bodies from just being a stiff. It gives us our movements, our personalities, our smile. You can be a person who is as dull as dishwater, just meandering through life, with very little life force. If you stayed physically healthy, your life force quotient would not matter. On the other hand, if you ended up with a disease like cancer, that quotient needs to be upgraded. Anyone who has seen another human or animal die has an understanding of life force.

I recall one of my flights back to the States from Vietnam. We had a passenger who was an officer in the Army who died of a heart attack while in mid flight. Our contract with the military stated that one crew member was to sit with the body until we arrived at our destination. That assignment went to the person lowest in seniority. At the time, that was me.

This had not been my first encounter with a dead person. As a child I had experienced several wakes displaying an open casket, including kissing the deceased person on the lips.

This flight was the first time that I spent any significant time with someone who had just recently died. The officer's body was covered with a blanket which made the experience a bit unsettling. For several hours after this man's death, his body went through rigor mortis, the progressive stiffening of his muscles.

Everytime his body moved, I moved. It was difficult not to think that at any moment, this man would throw the blanket off of his body and come alive, as I had seen him before his heart failure.

I sat with this corpse for 3 hours and tried to think of other thoughts, but my mind kept returning to the idea of life force. I was not calling it that at the time, but whatever the label, I was fascinated with the concept.

The only contact I had with this man was when I served him his dinner. He smiled briefly and he asked me for some water. In that short encounter, the connection I made with him was now enough to make me curious about his soul, his spirit or his life force. His voluntary and involuntary muscle movements, his smile, his voice - where did all of those things go after he died? What was really controlling them?

Those 3 hours gave me my first real education in life and death and one that I will never forget. Since that episode, I have spent hours wondering about the mortality of our souls. I have nothing profound to report, except that I have learned more about my soul and the souls of others, while experiencing life. What happens after death will remain a mystery until that moment. When that moment does come, we probably all hope that it will be with dignity and grace.

Everyone has a destiny, and no matter how much life force we generate, we will meet that destiny face to face. Might you believe that your destiny could be sabotaged or possibly *distracted?* Do you believe that you have the right to any and all information about treatments that may be less expensive, safer, nontoxic and possibly more successful than what is standard and *legal* in this country? Can and should we hold those people accountable who have forcibly prevented millions of Americans from having a choice in alternative treatments for cancer?

In my experience, alternative treatments for cancer are no less effective than the standard, conventional toxic treatments. Mainstream medicine adheres more to the politics of cancer and the "business" of health care (the $1-trillion-a-year health care in the United States!) than the therapies that are yet to be proven effective.

How can anybody call the treatments we standardly use for cancer a process toward healing? How can anybody heal in a hospital? If hospitals were truly healing places, then why do they have the lousiest food in town? You would never pay to eat at a restaurant what you receive for food in a hospital! You would complain to the manager and have a few choice words with the chef. Why don't hospitals have gardens where every day you experience fresh food, organically grown? What an example that would set for anyone coming to heal.

How about the lighting in a hospital? Or the colors or the chemicals used to clean the rooms of people already near death? Why is everyone wearing a white uniform? In some cultures, white symbolizes death. What is used to cover a person who dies in the hospital? A white sheet!

I have experienced a health care system that is NOT healthy, cost-*ineffective* and just plain toxic.

I have witnessed an organized medical monopoly around the field of cancer care in the United States that ensures a continuous flow of money to medical technology, research institutes and pharmaceutical companies. Do you realize how many millions of women, men and children have died of cancer in this century? How many of these deaths could have been prevented if instead of enforcing chemotherapy, radiation or surgery, these people had a choice of nontoxic treatments?

People insist on using war terminology to define the cancer experience or the losses involved. I could never agree with that. The "war" is not with the disease but with the politics of cancer.

As I participated as a civilian during my stint in Vietnam, I also now choose to remain a "civilian" in the war on or against cancer.

The only way any of us can deal with this crisis is to make our health our own business.

In the past four years, 500 people that I have interviewed have given me the faith to believe that with our destiny came many options. Each person with cancer took responsibility to learn when to strike or when to transform and shed their skin. No kin to a rattlesnake, but somewhere in the fear of this creature, each one imitated a rattler's tenacity. Find your "snake medicine" and like my buddy, Elvis says - FOCUS ON THE GOOD STUFF *ONLY!*

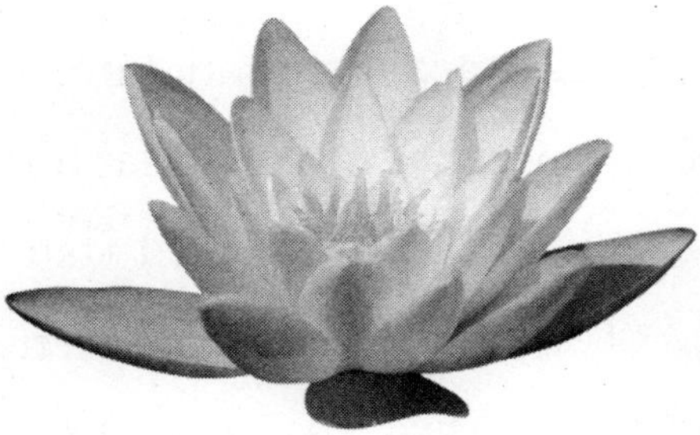

Some Final Words ...

Often I have been asked to tell someone "exactly everything" that I have done and continue to do to stay healthy. My reply is always the same. "I am not a guru. Do not follow me, you will only get lost."

This book is about finding *your* own personal way to healing. At first, that may disappoint you. I know how desperate people feel when their life or the life of a loved one is at stake. You must understand that if I tell you what I take each day or how much of something, then I should not be trusted. I have spent seventeen chapters extolling the importance of working with *your* immune system, *your* feelings, *your* type of disease - individually. Honor yourself or your loved one and seek your path.

It is truly not as difficult as you might think. People have told me that they wrote down the 15 Decisions and carried them wherever they went. When they started losing courage or their way, they would reread the decisions to bring them back.

If you are still not sure of your path or are feeling overwhelmed by your options, keep in mind that healing is a *process*. That process also extends into change. When we first hear that there are more options for treating cancer, we cannot imagine it to be true.

A man at one of my speeches told me that if that was true, "it would be on every billboard in the United States." How naive. He had never heard of anyone healing from cancer by choosing alternative treatments because of his lack of experience, and not because alternatives do not exist.

If you bought this book for someone who is skeptical, or you still feel that way, then ask yourself one last important question. Does your present treatment match up with your definition of healing?

Upon receiving a diagnosis of cancer, there is shock. One feels compelled to hang on to every word, every sentence, every sigh of their doctor. You want to trust your doctor and put your life in his experience.

After a period of time though, you may be perceptive enough to understand that your definition of "healing" is not matching the care you are receiving or the picture you see and feel around you. If it does not add up, that is your intuition calling. Pay attention, for it will not be long before you hear that voice more often.

Take the time to talk with people who have been through the same experience and have chosen different options. Be leery of computer data. Ask for names and phone numbers of others who have journeyed the same path. If you are told that they cannot supply such names because these people want to remain private, look for the door. In my experience, most people are very happy to talk about their experience, especially if they have benefited and are doing well. That is human nature.

Compliance with the 15 Decisions requires a new paradigm shift. A shift in the treatment of cancer and health care in general. Be open to it. I predict that in 10 years accepting the standard treatments for cancer will have vanished the way of the dinosaur. That is not such an outlandish prediction. The ground swell is already occurring. In the December issue of the *Journal of the American Medical Association,* a call was issued for published research papers on complementary medicine. Why is the AMA weakening its opposition to alternative medicine? Because the AMA cited the increased interest of its membership. Alternative medicine has become the No. 3 topic of interest among doctors and other readers of the journal. Last year it ranked 68th!

You do not need to wait for medical doctors to catch up. The train is leaving NOW! Trust your intuition and keep moving! This is YOUR LIFE, HEAL WITH IT!

RESOURCE GUIDE

INFORMATION SERVICES

Cancer Control Society, 2043 North Berendo St., Los Angeles,CA 90027, (213) 663-7801; Contact for extensive therapy information.

*The Health Resource,*209 Katherine Dr.,Conway, AZ. 72032, (501) 329-5272

International Health Information Institute, 14417 Chase St., Suite 432, Panorama City, CA. 91402

International Holistic Center, Inc., P.O. Box 15103, Phoenix, AZ. 85060, (602)957-3322

People Against Cancer, P.O. Box 10, Otho, IO 50569, (515) 972-4444

World Research Foundation, 15300 Ventura Blvd., Suite 405, Sherman Oaks, CA. 91403, (818) 907-5483

Cancer Treatment Centers of America, 2501 Emmaus Ave., Zion, Ill. 60099, 800-FOR-HELP.

EDUCATIONAL CENTERS - The following organizations offer information about specific therapies that they promote, as opposed to general information on cancer therapies.

Health Action, 19 East Mission St., Suite 102, Santa Barbara, CA.

93101, (805) 682-3230; Oriental medicine

Hippocrates Health Institute, 1443 Palmdale Ct.,West Palm Beach, FL 33411, (407) 471-8876; Nutrition

International Association for Oxygen Therapy, P.O.Box 1360, Priest River, ID 83856, (208)448-2504; Oxygen therapy

The Kushi Institute, P.O.Box 7, Beckett, MA 01223, (413) 623-5741; Macrobiotics

Optimum Health Institute of San Diego, 6970 Central Ave., Lemon Grove, CA 91945, (619) 464-3346; Nutrition

Linus Pauling Institute of Science and Medicine, 440 Page Mill Rd., Palo Alto,CA 94306, (415) 327-4064; Orthomolecular

Project Cure, 5910 North Central Expressway, Suite 760, Dallas,TX 75206, (214) 891-6111; Legal issues

Syracuse Cancer Research Institute, Inc., Presidential Plaza, 600 East Genesee St., Syracuse, N.Y. 13202, (315) 472-6616; Hydrazine sulfate

Ann Wigmore Foundation, 196 Commonwealth Ave., Boston, MA 02116, (617)267-9424; Nutrition

SUPPORT GROUPS

Cancer Self-Help Retreats, 2126 Green Hill Rd., Sebastopol, CA 95472, (800) 745-1837

Cancer Support Community, 401 Laurel St., San Francisco,CA 94118, (415)929-7400

Center For Attitudinal Healing, 19 Main St., Tiburon, CA. 94920, (415)435-5022

Colorado Outward Bound School, 945 Pennsylvania Ave., Denver, CO 80203, (303) 837-0880

Commonweal Cancer Help Program, P.O. Box 316, Bolinas, CA 94924, (415) 868-0970

Institute of Behavioral Medicine, 2200 Colorado Ave., Santa Monica, CA 90404, (310) 453-2300

Simonton Cancer Center, 15601 Sunset Blvd., Pacific Palisades, CA 90272, (310) 459-4434

TREATMENT CENTERS - Call the centers that interest you and ask for their information and names of patients who have attended these centers. Ask the patients about their experiences.

Livingston Foundation Medical Center, 3232 Duke St., San Diego, CA 92110, (619) 224-3515

Metabolic Clinic, Stanley Foster MD, 2810 Camino Del Rio S., #104, San Diego, CA 92108, (619) 543-9410

Burzynski Research Institute, (Antineoplaston Therapy), 12000 Richmond Ave., #260, Houston, TX 77082, (281) 597-0111

Immunology Researching Center, Lawrence Burton, PhD, Founder, Freeport Grand Bahamas Island, (US contact): P.O. Box 22579, Ft. Lauderdale, FL 33335, (242)352-7455

American Metabolic Institute, Geronimo Rubio MD, Tijuana,

Mexico (US contact): (800) 388-1083

American Biologics-Mexico S.A. Medical Center, 1180 Walnut Ave., Chula Vista, CA 91911 (619) 420-8200;

Health Restoration Center, 22706 Aspan St., Suite 501, Lake Forest, CA 92630, (714) 770-9616;

James Privitera MD, 105 N. Grandview Ave., Covina, CA 91723, (818) 966-1618

Davis Lamson,ND - Jonathan Wright MD, 515 W. Harrison St., #200, Kent,WA 98032, (206) 854-4900

Atkins Center for Complementary Medicine, 152 East 55th St., New York, NY 10022, (212) 758-2110

Nicholas Gonzalez MD, 737 Park Ave., New York, NY 10021 (212) 535-3993

Gerson Institute, Charlotte Gerson, Pres., P.O. Box 430, Bonita, CA 91908, (619) 585-7600

Gerson Therapy Self-Help, Marilyn Barnes, P.O. Box 16222, Oakland, CA 94610, (800) 851-8473

Max Gerson Memorial Cancer Center, Gar Hildenbrand, Pres., Gerson Research Organization, 7807 Artesian Rd., San Diego, CA 92127, (800) 759-2966

Helmut Keller MD, Chronic disease and Control Treatment Center, Am Reuthlein, 28675 Bad Steben, Germany, 011-49-9288-5167/66

Cancer Research Center, Ernesto Contreras, Jr. MD, Playas De Tijuana, Mexico, 011-52-66-809292, US contact: 539 Telegraph

Canyon Rd., #642, Chula Vista, CA 91910

Center for General Medicine and Acupuncture, Julian Mejia, MD, Tijuana, Mexico, (US contact) P.O. Box 2757, Chula Vista, CA 91212, (800) 390-5610

Hospital Santa Monica, Kurt Donsbach,Ph.D, Rosarita Beach, Mexico, 011-52-66-133333

Institute of Alternative Therapies, George Cardenas MD, Calle Penas, #1321 Secc. Jardines Del Sol, Playas De Tijuana, Mexico, 011-52-66-301232/301160

Douglas Brodie MD, 309 Kirman Ave., #2, Reno, NV 89502, (702) 324-7071

CANCER TESTS

American Medical Testing Labs, 1 Oakwood Blvd., #130, Hollywood, FL 33020, (800) 881-2685

Oncolab-AMAS Test, Samuel Bogoch MD,36 Fenway, Boston, MA 02215, (800) 922-8378

Healthexcel,(Nutritional Evaluation), P.O. Box 495, Winthrop, WA 98862, (509) 996-2131

LIVING WILLS

Five Wishes, Commission on Aging with Dignity, (888) -5-WISHES

Choice In Dying, 200 Varrick St., 10th Floor, NY, NY 10014-4810, (212) 366-5540

RIFE INSTRUMENT

Astropulse, 8690 Aero Dr., Ste.136, San Diego, CA 92129, (619)226-5050

HEALTHY READING

CONQUEST OF CANCER - Dr. Virginia Livingston

THE COOKBOOK (LIVINGSTON FOUNDATION) - Ana Maria Canalas

HEALTHY HEALING, A Guide to Self-Healing - Linda Rector Page, ND, PhD

THE ESSIAC REPORT - Richard Thomas

DETOXIFICATION AND HEALING, The Key To Optimal Health - Sidney MacDonald Baker, MD

ALTERNATIVE MEDICINE - THE DEFINITIVE GUIDE - The Burton Goldberg Group

DEFINITIVE GUIDE TO CANCER - John Diamond, MD and W. Lee Cowden,MD with Burton Goldberg

PRESCRIPTION FOR NUTRITIONAL HEALING - James F. Balch MD and Phyllis A. Balch, CNC

DR. WHITAKER'S GUIDE TO NATURAL HEALING - Julian Whitaker, MD

ENCYCLOPEDIA OF NUTRITIONAL SUPPLEMENTS - Michael T. Murray, ND

HERBAL DEFENSE - Positioning Yourself to Triumph Over Illness and Aging - Robyn Landis with Karta Purkh Singh Khalsa

OXYGEN HEALING THERAPIES - Nathaniel Altman

FULL CATASTROPHE LIVING: USING THE WISDOM OF YOUR BODY AND MIND TO FACE STRESS, PAIN AND ILLNESS - John Kabat-Zinn, PhD

THE 22 (NON-NEGOTIABLE) LAWS OF WELLNESS - Greg Anderson

REMARKABLE RECOVERY - Caryle Hirshberg and Marc Ian Barasch

CANCER THERAPY: THE INDEPENDENT CONSUMER'S GUIDE - Ralph W. Moss, PhD

COPING WITH PROSTATE CANCER - Robert H. Phillips, PhD

SPONTANEOUS HEALING - Andrew Weil, MD

HEALING WORDS:THE POWER OF PRAYER AND THE PRACTICE OF MEDICINE - Larry Dossey, MD

THIRD OPINION - John Fink

HEALING IMAGERY AND MUSIC -Carol A. Bush

SHARKS DON'T GET CANCER - Dr. I. William Lane

SMART MEDICINE FOR A HEALTHIER CHILD - Janet Zand, LAc and Rachel Walton, RN

ROYAL R. RIFE REPORT - Alison Davidson

OPTIONS: THE ALTERNATIVE CANCER THERAPY BOOK - Richard Walters

YOUR BODY BELIEVES EVERY WORD YOU SAY - Barbara Hoberman Levine

ORDER FORM

Please fill out the coupon below and mail it to:
Stray Dog Press
P.O.Box 1099
Calistoga, Ca. 94515
Or Call Toll Free: 1-888-322-8099

Please send me ___ copy(s) of CANCER THEN HEALING!

Name ______________________________________

Address ____________________________________

City_______________________ State_______ Zip _________

Number of Books____ @ $14.95 each = $_________

Add 7.25% sales tax to California addresses $_________

Shipping and Handling Charges@ $3.25 ea. book $_______

Total = $_______

Check____ Money Order____ Visa____ M/C____ AMEX____

Credit Card #_______________________ Exp. Date___ /___

Signature ___________________________________

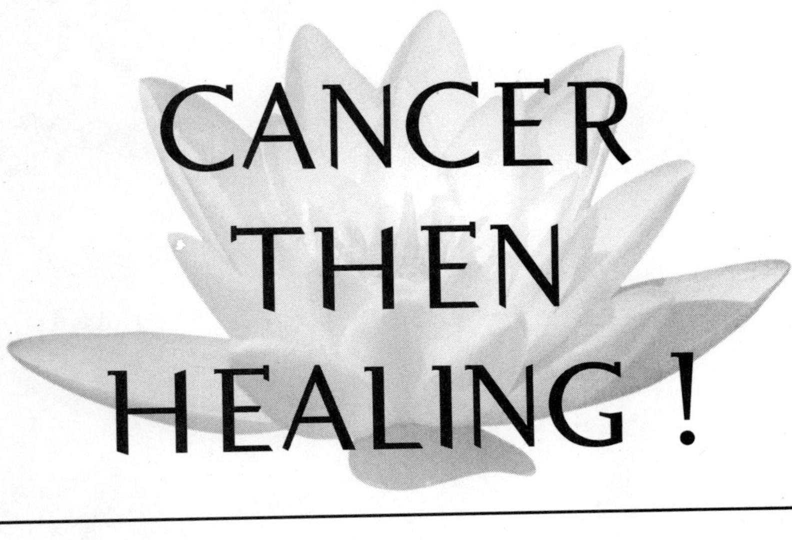